P9-APE-438

ROCKVILLE CAMPUS LIBRARY

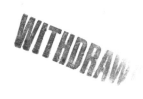

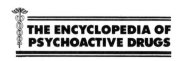

THE ENCYCLOPEDIA OF PSYCHOACTIVE DRUGS

IN 25 VOLUMES
Each title on a specific drug or drug-related problem

ALCOHOL
Alcohol And Alcoholism
Alcohol Customs & Rituals
Alcohol Teenage Drinking

HALLUCINOGENS
Flowering Plants Magic in Bloom
LSD Visions or Nightmares
Marijuana Its Effects on Mind & Body
Mushrooms Psychedelic Fungi
PCP The Dangerous Angel

NARCOTICS
Heroin The Street Narcotic
Methadone Treatment for Addiction
Prescription Narcotics The Addictive Painkillers

NON-PRESCRIPTION DRUGS
Over-the-Counter Drugs Harmless or Hazardous?

SEDATIVE HYPNOTICS
Barbiturates Sleeping Potion or Intoxicant?
Inhalants Glue, Gas & Sniff
Quaaludes The Quest for Oblivion
Valium The Tranquil Trap

STIMULANTS
Amphetamines Danger in the Fast Lane
Caffeine The Most Popular Stimulant
Cocaine A New Epidemic
Nicotine An Old-Fashioned Addiction

UNDERSTANDING DRUGS
The Addictive Personality
Escape from Anxiety and Stress
Getting Help Treatments for Drug Abuse
Treating Mental Illness
Teenage Depression and Drugs

METHADONE

WITHDRAWN

GENERAL EDITOR
Professor Solomon H. Snyder, M.D.
*Distinguished Service Professor of
Neuroscience, Pharmacology, and Psychiatry at
The Johns Hopkins University School of Medicine*

ASSOCIATE EDITOR
Professor Barry L. Jacobs, Ph.D.
Program in Neuroscience, Department of Psychology, Princeton University

---

SENIOR EDITORIAL CONSULTANT
Jerome H. Jaffe, M.D.
Director of The Addiction Research Center, National Institute on Drug Abuse

THE ENCYCLOPEDIA OF PSYCHOACTIVE DRUGS

METHADONE

Treatment for Addiction

WITHDRAWN

DONALD HUTCHINGS, Ph.D.

Columbia College of Physicians and Surgeons

1985
CHELSEA HOUSE PUBLISHERS
NEW YORK

SENIOR EDITOR: William P. Hansen
ASSOCIATE EDITORS: John Haney, Richard Mandell
CAPTIONS EDITOR: Richard Mandell
EDITORIAL COORDINATOR: Karyn Gullen Browne
ART DIRECTOR: Susan Lusk
LAYOUT: Carol McDougall
PICTURE RESEARCH: Susan Quist
COVER PHOTO: Frank Lusk

Copyright © 1985 by Chelsea House Publishers, a division of
Chelsea House Educational Communications, Inc. All rights reserved.
Printed and bound in the United States of America

First Printing

Library of Congress Cataloging in Publication Data
Hutchings, Donald.
    Methadone, treatment for addiction.
    (Encyclopedia of psychoactive drugs)
    Bibliography: p.
    Includes index.
    Summary: Discusses heroin addiction, its treatment
with methadone maintenance and alternatives, and other
aspects of modern drug abuse.
    1. Methadone maintenance—Juvenile literature. 2. Drug abuse—
Treatment—Juvenile literature.
[1. Methadone maintenance. 2. Heroin. 3. Drugs.
4. Drug abuse] I. Title. II. Series.
RC568.M4H88   1985   616.86′3   85-7915

ISBN 0-87754-760-2

Chelsea House Publishers
Harold Steinberg, Chairman & Publisher
Susan Lusk, Vice President
A Division of Chelsea House Educational Communications, Inc.

Chelsea House Publishers
133 Christopher Street
New York, NY 10014

Photos courtesy of AP/Wide World Photos, Eli Lilly Company, *High Times,*
National Library of Medicine, *Newsweek, The New York Times,* Phoenix House,
Rockefeller University, Roxanne Laboratories, Susan Quist, *Time,* UPI/Bettmann
Archive, and the Washington Post/D.C. Public Library.

CONTENTS

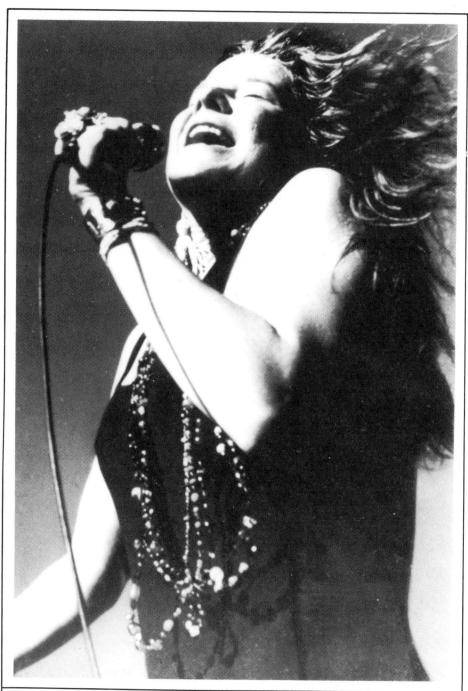

During the 1960s the emotional and exuberant Janis Joplin was the queen of rock 'n roll and blues. By 1970, after a controversial, fast-paced life, she was dead from an accidental overdose of heroin.

FOREWORD

In the Mainstream of American Life

The rapid growth of drug use and abuse is one of the most dramatic changes in the fabric of American society in the last 20 years. The United States has the highest level of psychoactive drug use of any industrialized society. It is 10 to 30 times greater than it was 20 years ago.

According to a recent Gallup poll, young people consider drugs the leading problem that they face. One of the legacies of the social upheaval of the 1960s is that psychoactive drugs have become part of the mainstream of American life. Schools, homes, and communities cannot be "drug proofed." There is a demand for drugs—and the supply is plentiful. Social norms have changed and drugs are not only available—they are everywhere.

Almost all drug use begins in the preteen and teenage years. These years are few in the total life cycle, but critical in the maturation process. During these years adolescents face the difficult tasks of discovering their identity, clarifying their sexual roles, asserting their independence, learning to cope with authority, and searching for goals that will give their lives meaning. During this intense period of growth, conflict is inevitable and the temptation to use drugs is great. Drugs are readily available, adolescents are curious and vulnerable, there is peer pressure to experiment, and there is the temptation to escape from conflicts.

No matter what their age or socioeconomic status, no group is immune to the allure and effects of psychoactive drugs. The U.S. Surgeon General's report, "Healthy People," indicates that 30% of all deaths in the United States

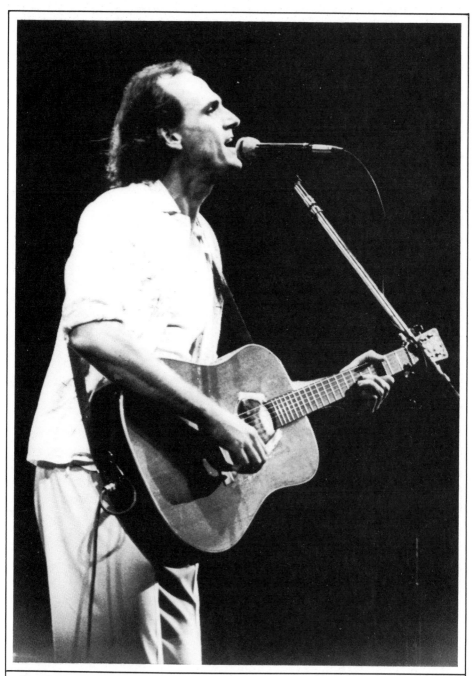

***Previous to methadone treatment, song writer and musician James Taylor
described himself as having the "tendency to crawl into a hole and poison
myself." When treatment ended in 1974 he said, "I like to think that this is
the point at which I finally get off the cycle."***

are premature because of alcohol and tobacco use. However, the most shocking development in this report is that mortality in the age group between 15 and 24 has increased since 1960 despite the fact that death rates for all other age groups have declined in the 20th century. Accidents, suicides, and homicides are the leading cause of death in young people 15 to 24 years of age. In many cases the deaths are directly related to drug use.

THE ENCYCLOPEDIA OF PSYCHOACTIVE DRUGS answers the questions that young people are likely to ask about drugs, as well as those they might not think to ask, but should. Topics include: what it means to be intoxicated; how drugs affect mood; why people take drugs; who takes them; when they take them; and how much they take. They will learn what happens to a drug when it enters the body. They will learn what it means to get "hooked" and how it happens. They will learn how drugs affect their driving, their schoolwork, and those around them—their peers, their family, their friends, and their employers. They will learn what the signs are that indicate that a friend or a family member may have a drug problem and to identify four stages leading from drug use to drug abuse. Myths about drugs are dispelled.

National surveys indicate that students are eager for information about drugs and that they respond to it. Students not only need information about drugs—they want information. How they get it often proves crucial. Providing young people with accurate knowledge about drugs is one of the most critical aspects.

THE ENCYCLOPEDIA OF PSYCHOACTIVE DRUGS synthesizes the wealth of new information in this field and demystifies this complex and important subject. Each volume in the series is written by an expert in the field. Handsomely illustrated, this multi-volume series is geared for teenage readers. Young people will read these books, share them, talk about them, and make more informed decisions because of them.

Miriam Cohen, Ph.D.
Contributing Editor

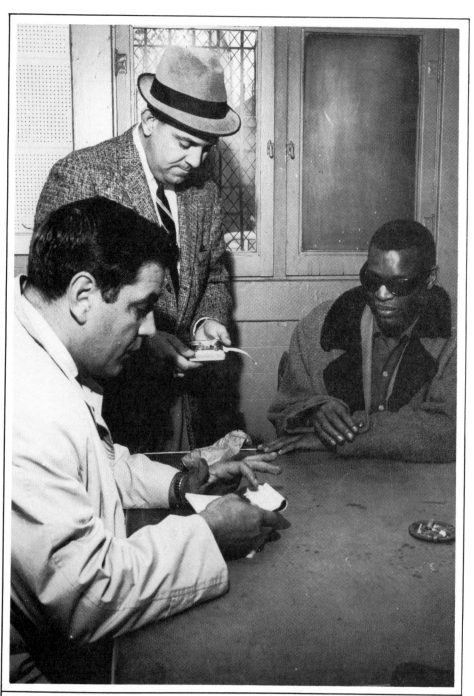

In 1961 singer and musician Ray Charles, then one of America's top recording stars, was arrested on a narcotics charge after police seized opiates and related paraphernalia from his Indianapolis hotel room.

INTRODUCTION

The Gift of Wizardry
Use and Abuse

JACK H. MENDELSON, M.D.
NANCY K. MELLO, PH.D.
Alcohol and Drug Abuse Research Center
Harvard Medical School—McLean Hospital

Dorothy to the Wizard:

"I think you are a very bad man," said Dorothy.
"Oh, no, my dear; I'm really a very good man; but I'm a very bad Wizard."
—from THE WIZARD OF OZ

Man is endowed with the gift of wizardry, a talent for discovery and invention. The discovery and invention of substances that change the way we feel and behave are among man's special accomplishments, and like so many other products of our wizardry, these substances have the capacity to harm as well as to help. The substance itself is neutral, an intricate molecular structure. Yet, "too much" can be sickening, even deadly. It is man who decides how each substance is used, and it is man's beliefs and perceptions that give this neutral substance the attributes to heal or destroy.

Consider alcohol—available to all and yet regarded with intense ambivalence from biblical times to the present day. The use of alcoholic beverages dates back to our earliest ancestors. Alcohol use and misuse became associated with the worship of gods and demons. One of the most powerful Greek gods was Dionysus, lord of the Underworld and god of wine. The Romans adopted Dionysus but changed his name to Bacchus. Festivals and holidays associated with Bacchus celebrated the harvest and the origins of life. Time has blurred the images of the Bacchanalian festival, but the theme of drunkenness as a major part of celebration has survived the pagan gods and remains a familiar part of modern society. The term "Bacchanalian festival" conveys a more appealing image than "drunken orgy" or "pot

13

party," but whatever the label, some of the celebrants will inevitably start up the "high" escalator to the next plateau. Once there, the de-escalation is difficult for many.

According to reliable estimates, one out of every ten Americans develops a serious alcohol-related problem sometime in his or her lifetime. In addition, automobile accidents caused by drunken drivers claim the lives of tens of thousands every year. Many of the victims are gifted young people, just starting out in adult life. Hospital emergency rooms abound with patients seeking help for alcohol-related injuries.

Who is to blame? Can we blame the many manufacturers who produce such an amazing variety of alcoholic beverages? Should we blame the educators who fail to explain the perils of intoxication, or so exaggerate the dangers of drinking that no one could possibly believe them? Are friends to blame—those peers who urge others to "drink more and faster," or the macho types who stress the importance of being able to "hold your liquor"? Casting blame, however, is hardly constructive, and pointing the finger is a fruitless way to deal with problems. Alcoholism and drug abuse have few culprits but many victims. Accountability begins with each of us, every time we choose to use or to misuse an intoxicating substance.

It is ironic that some of man's earliest medicines, derived from natural plant products, are used today to poison and to intoxicate. Relief from pain and suffering is one of society's many continuing goals. Over 3,000 years ago, the Therapeutic Papyrus of Thebes, one of our earliest written records, gave instructions for the use of opium in the treatment of pain. Opium, in the form of its major derivative, morphine, remains one of the most powerful drugs we have for pain relief. But opium, morphine, and similar compounds, such as heroin, have also been used by many to induce changes in mood and feeling. Another example of man's misuse of a natural substance is the coca leaf, which for centuries was used by the Indians of Peru to reduce fatigue and hunger. Its modern derivative, cocaine, has important medical use as a local anesthetic. Unfortunately, its increasing abuse in the 1980s has reached epidemic proportions.

The purpose of this series is to provide information about the nature and behavioral effects of alcohol and drugs, and the probable consequences of both their moderate use and abuse. The authors believe that up-to-date, objective information about alcohol and drugs will help readers make better decisions as to whether to use them or not. The information presented here (and in other books in this series) is based on many clinical and laboratory studies and observations by people from diverse walks of life.

Over the centuries, novelists, poets, and dramatists have provided us with many insights into the beneficial and problematic aspects of alcohol and drug use. Physicians, lawyers, biologists, psychologists, and social scientists have contributed to a better understanding of the causes and consequences of using these substances. The authors in this series have attempted to gather and condense all the latest information about drug use and abuse. They have also described the sometimes wide gaps in our knowledge and have suggested some new ways to answer many difficult questions.

One such question, for example, is how do alcohol and drug problems get started? And what is the best way to treat them when they do? Not too many years ago, alcoholics and drug abusers were regarded as evil, immoral, or both. It is now recognized that these persons suffer from very complicated diseases involving deep psychological and social problems. To understand how the disease begins and progresses, it is necessary to understand the nature of the substance, the behavior of the afflicted person, and the characteristics of the society or culture in which he lives.

The diagram below shows the interaction of these three factors. The arrows indicate that the substance not only affects the user personally, but the society as well. Society influences attitudes towards the substance, which in turn affect its availability. The substance's impact upon the society may support or discourage the use and abuse of that substance.

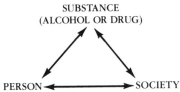

SUBSTANCE
(ALCOHOL OR DRUG)

PERSON ⟷ SOCIETY

Although many of the social environments we live in are very similar, some of the most subtle differences can strongly influence our thinking and behavior. Where we live, go to school and work, whom we discuss things with—all influence our opinions about drug use and misuse. Yet we also share certain commonly accepted beliefs that outweigh any differences in our attitudes. The authors in this series have tried to identify and discuss the central, most crucial issues concerning drug use and misuse.

Regrettably, man's wizardry in developing new substances in medical therapeutics has not always been paralleled by intelligent usage. Although we do know a great deal about the effects of alcohol and drugs, we have yet to learn how to impart that knowledge, especially to young adults.

Does it matter? What harm does it do to smoke a little pot or have a few beers? What is it like to be intoxicated? How long does it last? Will it make me feel really fine? Will it make me sick? What are the risks? These are but a few of the questions answered in this series, which, hopefully, will enable the reader to make wise decisions concerning the crucial issue of drugs.

Information sensibly acted upon can go a long way towards helping everyone develop his or her best self. As one keen and sensitive observer, Dr. Lewis Thomas, has said,

> "There is nothing at all absurd about the human condition. We matter. It seems to me a good guess, hazarded by a good many people who have thought about it, that we may be engaged in the formation of something like a mind for the life of this planet. If this is so, we are still at the most primitive stage, still fumbling with language and thinking, but infinitely capacitated for the future. Looked at this way, it is remarkable that we've come as far as we have in so short a period, really no time at all as geologists measure time. We are the newest, the youngest, and the brightest thing around."

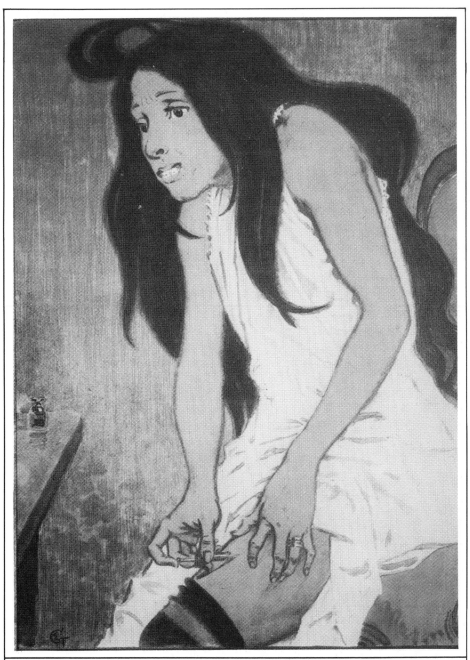

Heroin users, desperate to break their drug habits, fill treatment centers beyond capacity. Because of this many addicts have been turned away, forced to return to the streets. In 1981 there were 1360 narcotic deaths reported to DAWN (the Drug Abuse Warning Network). Thirteen of these were youths between the ages of 10 and 17.

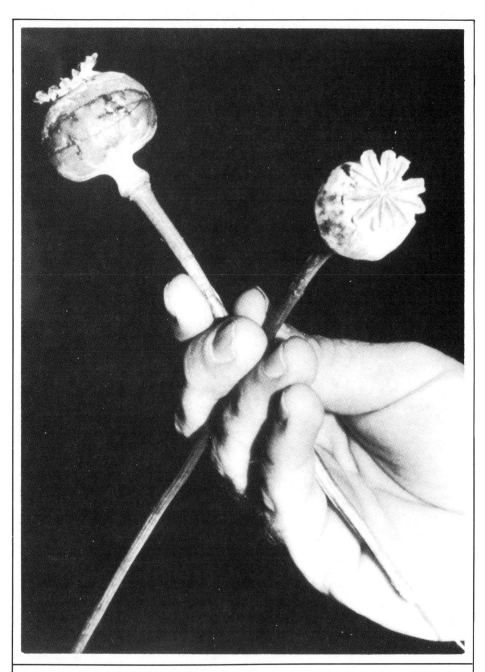

Opium is harvested from the poppy, Papaver somniferum, *just after the petals fall. The unripened seed capsules, above, are incised and an alkaloid seeps out which, within 24 hours, dries to a gum. Even when lanced several times each capsule releases very little opium. It takes nearly 3,000 poppies to create 3.5 pounds of opium.*

CHAPTER 1

HISTORY OF THE OPIATES

Methadone is a drug used to treat heroin addiction, and, along with heroin and morphine, is a member of the family of drugs called the *opiates.* All the opiates share unique characteristics, both with respect to their origin and to the effects they have on the human body. They are among the most effective drugs known for the alleviation of pain and other serious discomforts. However, they can produce an addiction that is so seductive and overpowering that individuals will do almost anything—steal, murder, lie, prostitute themselves, or risk life and limb—to ensure a continuous supply of the drug.

In order to better understand methadone, its relationship to the other opiates, and its own use and properties, it is necessary to gain a historical perspective. The history of the use and abuse of the opiates is long and complex, spanning centuries of problems which involve social-class attitudes and prejudices, economic and legal issues, as well as international power politics. While entire volumes and monographs have been devoted to describing these events, this short introduction will highlight the most important developments.

Early "Aspirin"

Opiates come from the milky juice of the poppy plant, *Papaver somniferum*. (The term opium comes from the Greek word for vegetable juice.) There are written references to poppy juice that can be traced back to the third century B.C. Arabian physicians were familiar with the medicinal uses of opium, and in the seventh century A.D. Arabian traders introduced it to the Orient, where it came to be used to treat pain and diarrhea. By the 16th century the medicinal use of opium was well known in Europe, and in 1680 it was written, "Among the remedies which it has pleased almighty God to give to man to relieve his sufferings, none is so universal and so efficacious as opium."

In England, during the 1800s opium was freely available and could be purchased at the grocery store. People in the working class were using opium as a cheap alternative to beer, and it was even sold in pubs or added directly to beer. But eventually problems with its use began to be

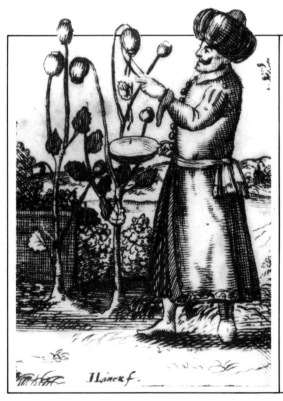

In a 1674 etching a man in Eastern dress stands in a garden as he slashes an opium seed capsule. Small ceramic jugs, created in the shape of poppies and discovered in Cyprus, prove that opium, dissolved in water or wine, was being exported to Egypt as early as 1500 B.C. And it was not long before Egypt too was cultivating the poppy.

noticed. Preparations which contained opiates could be linked to an increasing number of both infant and adult deaths. This, along with the rising incidence of drug-related crime, led to the legal restrictions of its sale and use in England in 1868.

During the 19th century, in the United States the opium poppy was grown in New England and in the South, though most of what was used for the manufacture of heroin and morphine was imported. It was the "aspirin" of the times and was inexpensive and easily obtained. Opiates were generously dispensed by physicians and were available from groceries, general stores, pharmacies, and mail-order companies. At this time there were approximately 600 opiate-based, nonprescription medicines available and sold as infant teething syrups, pain-killers, cough mixtures, and "women's friends." Billboards and magazines advertised such opium-containing products as Ayer's Cherry Pectoral, Mrs. Winslow's Soothing Syrup, and McMunn's Elixir of Opium.

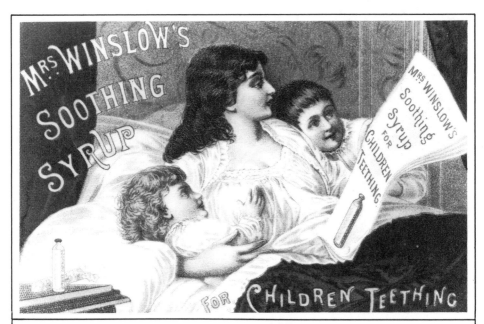

After morphine ($C_1H_{19}NO_3$), opium's principal active ingredient, was isolated by a German pharmacist in 1815, it was included in many remedies, such as Mrs. Winslow's Soothing Syrup for teething.

But to understand the reason for the popularity of opium, it must be noted that effective alternatives to its use were not yet available. There was no Kaopectate to treat simple diarrhea, or aspirin to alleviate the minor discomforts of headache, arthritis, or menstrual cramps. Babies frequently died from gastrointestinal disorders unless treated with opium. And while there was no adequate treatment for the common and often fatal tuberculosis, relief from some of its symptoms, such as the debilitating, hacking cough, could be alleviated with opiates.

Though the use of opiates for these various maladies was totally accepted, nonmedical use, both in England and the United States, was scorned as a depraved, immoral vice, equal to the excessive use of alcohol. However, in the 19th century opium was as legal as beer, and though its use was disapproved, so-called "opium-eaters" (the terms addict and addiction had not yet come into use) were not subject to

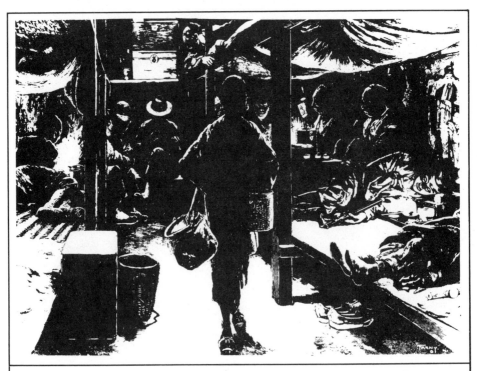

In the late 19th century underground opium dens, such as the one seen here in a 1888 lithograph by H.F. Farny, dotted San Francisco.

the severe moral sanctions associated with opium use today. Regular users were generally not fired from their jobs or divorced by their spouses, nor were their children removed to foster homes. In fact they typically continued to participate as normal members of their community, workplace, and family. Opiates, though socially unacceptable, were not considered a menace to society.

Opium Dens

A historical recounting of the opiates would not be complete without mentioning the opium dens. During the 1850s and 1860s tens of thousands of Chinese entered the United States to become part of the cheap labor force which built the great Western railroads. And with them they brought the practice of opium smoking. Confined mostly to the western part of the United States, opium smoking was an integral part of the Chinese lifestyle, and was engaged in

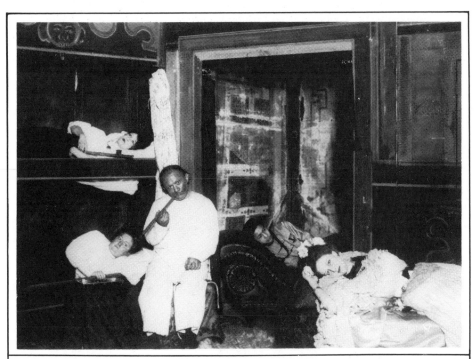

Soon after their appearance in San Francisco, opium dens could be found in most U.S. cities. Here, in 1926 opium is smoked in a New York den in the same manner as did people in Cyprus in the 12th century B.C.

largely as a relaxing and pleasurable pastime. Though we are now aware of opium's addictive qualities and would be naive to assume that during this period there was no compulsive use, it seems that most smoked only recreationally. Typically it was smoked at the end of the work day, either in the bunk house of a remote work area or in an opium den located in a nearby large city. This practice is quite similar to the custom of contemporary westerners who after work congregate in the local bar or tavern to drink and socialize with friends. But soon Caucasian men and even greater numbers of Caucasian women "from respectable families" began the practice of smoking opium, and the authorities blamed the "heathen" Chinese for corrupting their morals. Local ordinances—the first appearing in San Francisco in 1875—threatened users with fines and imprisonment, but failed to curb the use of opium despite the subsequent enactment of even more severe penalties. In 1909 a federal law was enacted which prohibited the importation of opium for smoking. Even stricter laws were still to come. Yet opium dens could be found in most major cities as recently as in the 1930s.

Morphine and the Hypodermic Syringe

During the last quarter of the 19th century opiates were ingested principally by eating opium or drinking liquid preparations of morphine. However, abuse of alcohol was at that

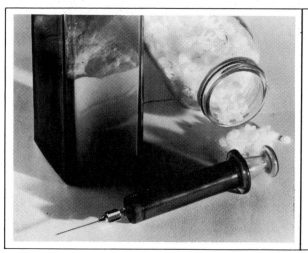

The hypodermic needle, invented in 1853, provided a quick route to the morphine and heroin euphoria. First made of glass and hardened steel, the needle could be repeatedly used by both doctors and addicts.

time still of much greater social concern than the abuse of opiates. But several developments occurred during the century which led to the emergence of an opiate addiction problem.

In 1803 a substance was isolated from crude opium and identified as one of the major active ingredients. It was named morphine, after Morpheus, the Greek god of dreams. Then, in 1853 the hypodermic syringe was invented. By the middle of the century the use of pure morphine, rather than crude opium preparations, had become common throughout

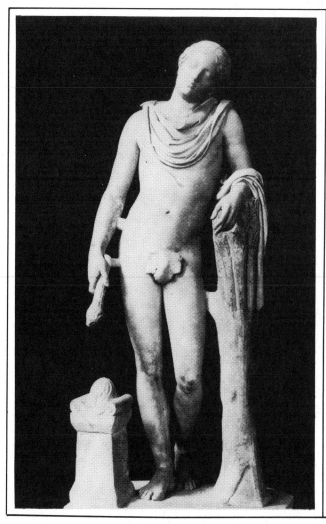

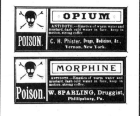

Because of the drug's sedative qualities, morphine was named after Morpheus, the Greek god of dreams represented in this statue. In 1906, when outcry over spreading addiction grew loud enough, manufacturers were required by law to attach labels, such as those above, to all their opium-containing products. The antidotes, however, reflect turn-of-the-century ignorance of the severity and complexity of these dangerous drugs.

the medical world. Both the availability of morphine and the ability to inject the drug directly into the body marked a critical turning point. The large-scale medical use of injected morphine to treat the wounded of the Civil War was one of several developments that contributed to a growing epidemic of compulsive opiate use. A substantial number of those addicted were physicians and other professionals who had ready access to the drug and the syringe. Along with the availability of opiate-based nonprescription medicines, all these events led to the creation of an addiction problem which peaked during the 1890s.

Congress Acts — The Law Steps In

In response to an intense public outcry at the growing menace of "dope fiends" and "opium-eaters," in 1906 Congress passed the first Pure Food and Drug Act, which re-

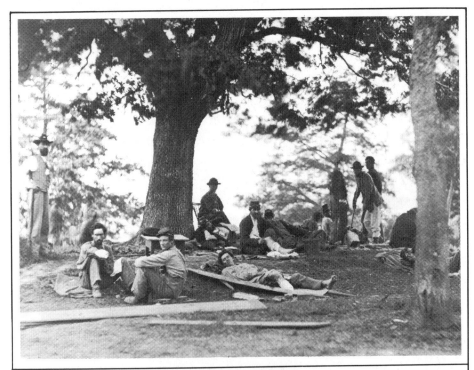

Morphine was widely used during the Civil War to treat wounded soldiers such as these left in the field after the Battle of Chancellorsville.

quired manufacturers to label those nonprescription medicines that contained opiates. In addition, at this time there were also educational campaigns that warned of the dangers of addiction from opium-based medicines. As a result, up until 1914 there appeared to be a modest decline in addiction. But the legislation and educational programs had little direct impact on those already addicted and, most importantly, did not cut off their legal supply of the drug.

In 1914 Congress passed the Harrison Narcotic Act, which provided for the taxation and orderly marketing of opiates and certain other drugs. Only small quantities were allowed in over-the-counter preparations, and larger quantities could be obtained only through a physician's prescription. As a result, the availability of legal opiates was severely curtailed. The amount of opiates permitted in nonprescription medicines was reduced to a level so low that they became nonaddicting. But these same medicines also afforded little or no relief for the individual already addicted.

Since opiate addiction was considered a moral problem rather than a disease, as it is now, law enforcement officers considered physicians to be in violation of the law if they prescribed opiates for an addict. And, in fact, many were arrested, and some convicted and imprisoned. Thus, addicts, some of whom did not even realize they had become dependent on their medicine, were abruptly cut off from their legal supply of the drug and had no recourse to medical treatment. The results were swift, predictably tragic, and best conveyed in reactions from the medical community.

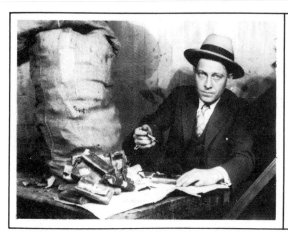

By 1924 the U.S. Narcotic Division in San Francisco had collected 2,500 cans of narcotics, most of it opium. Here an agent examines opium prior to burning it in the furnace.

In May 1915, a mere six weeks after the effective date of the Harrison Act, an editorial in the *New York Medical Journal* declared:

> *As was expected ... the immediate effects of the Harrison antinarcotic law were seen in the flocking of drug habitués to hospitals and sanitoriums. Sporadic crimes of violence were reported too, due usually to desperate efforts by addicts to obtain drugs, but occasionally to a delirious state induced by sudden withdrawal. ...*
>
> *The really serious results of this legislation, however, will only appear gradually and will not always be recognized as such. These will be the failures of promising careers, the disrupting of happy families, the commission of crimes which will never be traced to their real cause, and the influx into hospitals for the mentally disordered of many who would otherwise live socially competent lives.*

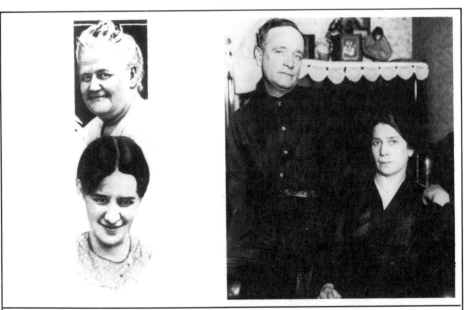

In 1923 opiate addicts Ella Woolson (top left) and her daughter Edna (bottom left) committed suicide when told that the cure would separate them. They were discovered by Ella's son, William, and his wife.

A few months later, an editorial in *American Medicine* read:

> *Abuses in the sale of narcotic drugs are increasing. . . . A particular sinister sequence. . .is the character of the places to which [addicts] are forced to go to get their drugs and the type of people with whom they are obliged to mix. The most depraved criminals are often the dispensers of these habit forming drugs. The moral dangers, as well as the effect on the self-respect of the addict, call for no comment. One has only to think of the stress under which the addict lives, and to recall his lack of funds, to realize the extent to which these . . . afflicted individuals are under the control of the worst elements of society. In respect to female habitués the conditions are worse, if possible. Houses of ill repute are usually their source of supply, and one has only to think of what repeated visitations to such places mean to countless good women and girls— unblemished in most instances except for an unfortunate addiction to some narcotic drug—to appreciate the terrible menace.*

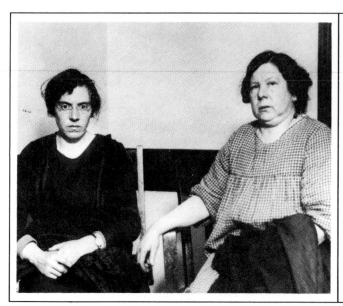

The smuggling of drugs has never been limited only to tough underworld figures. In 1924 the two women pictured here, nurses on the S.S. America, were arrested with narcotics valued at $75,000.

In 1918 a congressional committee investigated the problem and among the conclusions reported the following:

> *Opiates, cocaine, and other drugs were being used by about a million people.*
>
> *The "underground" traffic in narcotic drugs was about equal to the legitimate medical traffic.*
>
> *The "dope peddlers" appeared to have established a national organization, smuggling drugs through seaports or across the Canadian and Mexican borders.*
>
> *The illicit use of narcotics has actually increased since the passage of the Harrison Act. The increases occurred in the large cities, a likely result of addicts migrating to major metropolitan areas where black markets in heroin and many other illicit drugs flourish.*

The Effects of Harsher Laws

The failure of the Harrison Act to stem the addiction problem or curb the black market did not, however, lead to any change in policy. Rather, a series of newer and stricter

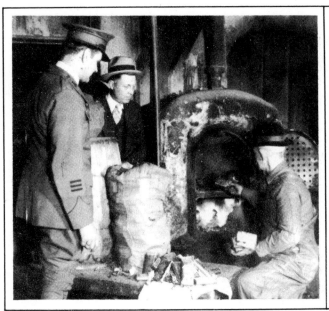

On January 23, 1926, this stash of opium, morphine, and cocaine valued at $250,000 ceased to be a menace to the world and a worry to customs officials when it was tossed into an incinerator.

laws providing for increasingly longer maximum sentences were enacted. Many states steadily increased the original two years maximum imprisonment until the penalty was life sentence without probation. Finally, during the 1950s federal and some state antinarcotic laws included the death penalty. Yet the enactment of these stiffer penalties left the problem relatively unchanged.

There are now approximately one-half million opiate addicts—an estimated 190,000 in the New York City metropolitan area alone—and a flourishing multi-billion-dollar international market in illicit drugs, whose profits match those of many of our largest corporations. In the 1980s the great American disease has never been more firmly entrenched. But unlike the problem at the turn of the century, instead of housewives drinking morphine elixirs, or artists and writers smoking opium, now a deviant subculture made up of people from all social classes—from the poor and disadvantaged to middle- and upper-class affluent professionals—is injecting heroin.

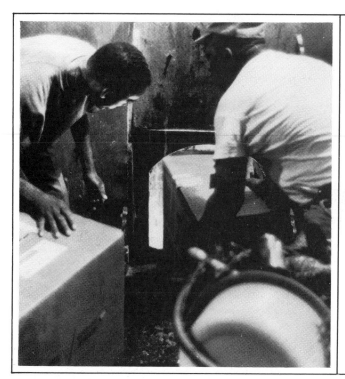

Seized narcotics being burned in 1926. In 1983 illicit opium production, most of which was converted to heroin, may have been as high as 2,000 tons. According to the Drug Enforcement Administration four tons of heroin are smuggled into the U.S. each year.

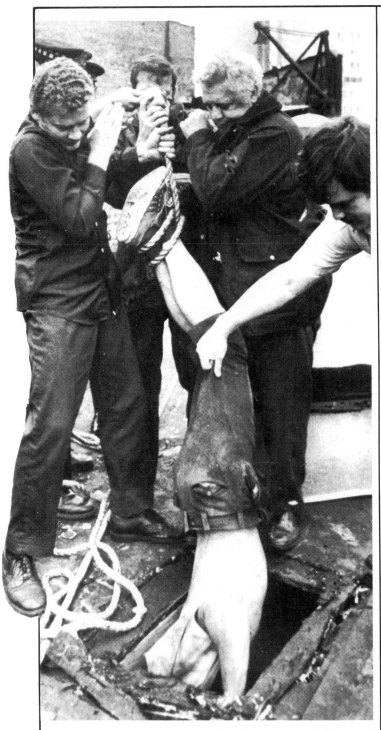

Addicts will often go to any means to secure their fix. In an attempt to rob a Chicago drug store, a 27-year-old man slid down an air-conditioning duct. Unfortunately for him, the duct proved to be too narrow. After six hours of being trapped between four metal walls, police and firemen were able to hoist him out. He was charged with burglary.

CHAPTER 2

GETTING HOOKED ON HEROIN

I started messing with drugs when I was 15. It was the last day of school and a friend gave me a snort of heroin. 'Take a blow, you're going to love the high,' she told me. And she was right. When I was 17, I dropped out of high school and got a job in the post office. I worked there for about a year when I found another way of making money—bagging heroin. You can make about $100 a day in one of the mills. And the bosses always have some cocaine to keep you perky and to stop you from dozing off because of the heroin fumes.

"It's hard to get those jobs in the mills and it costs me $100 to $150 a week to get heroin. I'm on welfare but that's not enough. I get money in various ways, sell pills, make a heroin run for someone else and get paid by the customer. The one thing I won't do is prostitute myself. I also won't sell drugs to any children. I've only been arrested once. I was with three other people when the cops caught us shooting up in a hallway. I've tried going cold turkey but it doesn't work. I have a lot of problems, pressures, finding enough money to raise my kids. If I can't handle something, I have to get high. It takes the tension off me."

(Told by a 35-year-old woman who has two children and has always lived in Harlem, a black ghetto in New York City.)

"I come from a good family. My father was a postman, my brothers and sisters all have good jobs. When I was 13, a friend had some heroin. He asked if anyone wanted to get high. It was a big thing back then. I said, 'I'll try.' I main-lined and I've been screwing up ever since.

"My parents were immigrants. They didn't know any-thing about drugs and they didn't realize I was screwing around until I got arrested for burglary when I was 16. All in all, I spent about 10 years in prison for robberies and burglaries. I used to push drugs and I made $1,000 a week. But I would spend it all on heroin. I'm married and have two sons, 12 and 7. My wife doesn't know what I'm doing. I never go into the house high. She thinks I'm straight and that I'm a cabby.

"I got out of prison about a year ago, after four years of armed robbery. Heroin is costing me about $60 a day. I'm shooting five or six bags. To pay for it, I pull a job once a week, usually a stickup. Most of the time I don't know what I'm doing. I wake up and find I have $3,000 or $4,000 in my pocket. Then the picture would come back to me that I stuck somebody up.

"My parole officer never looks at my arms. He asks if I'm working and says keep looking. They don't care as long as you come in and keep the appointments. It's a bitch out there getting a job. Certain jobs you have to be bonded. With my record, I can't even get a super's job. I want to stop but I don't know how. It's hell out there. I get so depressed that instead of looking for a job, I buy a bag of that poison."

(Told by a 35-year-old white male who grew up in a working-class Italian neighborhood in New York City.*)

Addicts and Addiction

The term addiction, because of popular usage, has taken on a variety of meanings. "Football widows" complain that their husbands are addicted to the sport, while others describe themselves as addicted to a particular brand or flavor of ice cream, type of candy bar, or even a certain TV show. In such contexts addiction is used to characterize behavior that ranges from an occasional preoccupation to a continuous, obsessive involvement with some substance or activity. Such a description appears to characterize behavior associated

---

*From interviews published in a series in *The New York Times*, May 20–24, 1984.

with drug abuse, but because of the term's broad meaning it lacks precision. More importantly, its common usage fails to include the process of tolerance, or distinguish psychological from physical dependence. As will be shown, such a distinction is necessary for an understanding of the effects of opiates, particularly when compared to other substances of abuse.

Scientifically, the term addiction is defined as a behavioral pattern of drug use characterized by an overwhelming, compulsive involvement with its use and the securing of its supply, and a high tendency to relapse after withdrawal.

How the Opiates Make You Feel

Heroin, methadone, and the other opiates produce effects on a variety of organs and bodily processes, but because we are mainly concerned with the abuse of heroin and its treatment with methadone, this discussion will be confined to the effects of opiates on the brain. It is here where the opiates are most powerful and produce their dramatic effects on pain and mood. And it is also in the brain where the events that lead to addiction and withdrawal occur.

When heroin and related opioids are introduced into the body they produce analgesia (a reduction in pain sensitivity), decrease sexual drive, reduce aggression, and cause drowsiness, changes in mood, and mental clouding. Nonad-

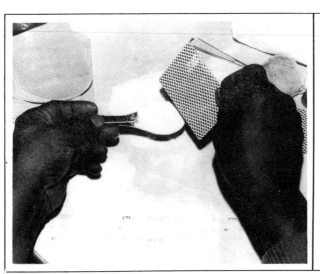

Though the rituals surrounding drug use are often elaborate, the paraphernalia is generally quite crude and unsterile. Here an addict measures a heroin mixture with a tablespoon and levels it with a playing card.

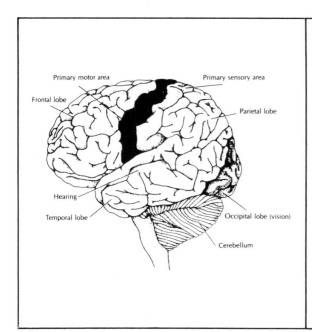

Primary motor area
Frontal lobe
Primary sensory area
Parietal lobe
Hearing
Temporal lobe
Occipital lobe (vision)
Cerebellum

Figure 1. *Research has discovered that the brain itself produces morphine-like substances called endorphins, which, when attached to the opium-receptors located in the brain, alleviate pain and fear. Morphine's similarity to the endorphins enables it to fit into these same receptors and produce identical effects.*

dicted individuals may also experience euphoria and a care-free sense of well-being, whereas some experience unpleasant effects such as nausea, vomiting, drowsiness, the inability to concentrate, slowed thinking, and lethargy. The strength of these effects is determined by how much of the drug reaches the brain, which, in turn, depends on how it is introduced into the body.

When taken orally, opiates are rapidly metabolized, or broken down, by the liver so that only a small amount reaches the brain. When administered intravenously the drug immediately enters the blood, and the liver is initially by-passed. Within seconds a significant amount of the drug goes directly to the brain to produce its potent effects. The effects are instantaneous and powerful—a warm flushing of the skin and a pleasant feeling in the pit of the stomach, which addicts liken to a sexual orgasm. These sensations, referred to as a "rush," "kick," or "bang," last about 45 seconds and are followed by an overall feeling of well-being, tranquillity, and dreamy indifference. Thus, because of this great difference in time of onset of the effects, the addict generally prefers to inject or "mainline" heroin rather than take it by mouth.

Developing Tolerance

In response to repeated and regular exposure to any of the opiates, the body develops a steadily increasing capacity or tolerance. This is an indication that the body, or more accurately, certain physiological processes, have adapted to the presence of the drug and no longer respond as strongly as before. Thus, if the same dose is taken daily, the effects produced on the body diminish.

As tolerance develops, in order to produce the same effect increasingly larger doses of the drug are required, and thus the heroin user will have to take larger doses of heroin each day to experience the same effects as when the addiction first started. Therefore, what begins as a $10-a-day habit soon escalates to a $100-a-day habit as more and more of

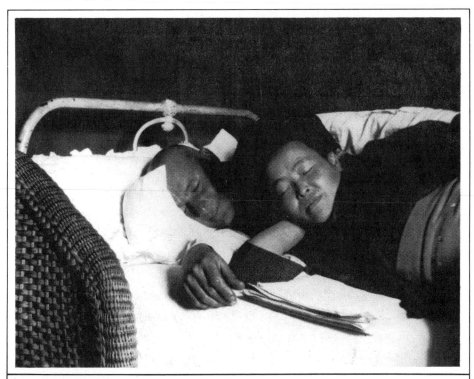

By the 17th century opium was being smoked in China. Here, in Shanghai in 1921, a Chinese couple, after using opium, sleeps peacefully. Opiate use produces both euphoria and drowsiness.

the drug is needed. In addition, cross-tolerance develops. This means that an individual who has developed tolerance to heroin will also show tolerance to morphine or methadone. Because of this characteristic, tolerance to heroin also results in increased doses of other opiates.

Dependence and Withdrawal

Along with tolerance, another process occurs—the development of physical dependence. As the body adapts to the presence of the drug it comes to depend on its presence in order to function normally. When deprived of its daily dose, a state of opiate withdrawal or abstinence occurs. In many respects withdrawal effects are the opposite of those produced by the drug—tranquillity is replaced with torment, relaxation with excitement, euphoria with restlessness, and calm serenity with agitated depression.

The character and severity of the withdrawal symptoms that appear when an opioid is discontinued depend upon many factors, including the type of drug, the total daily dose, the interval between doses, the duration of use, and the health and personality of the addict.

In the case of morphine or heroin, excessive tearing of the eyes, running nose, yawning, and perspiration appear during withdrawal. The addict may fall into a restless sleep that may last several hours but from which he or she awakens more restless and miserable than before.

Symptoms increase and become progressively more severe—dilated pupils, loss of appetite, gooseflesh, restlessness, irritability, and tremors. With symptoms reaching their peak at about 48 to 72 hours after the last dose of opiate, the addict shows increasing irritability, insomnia, complete loss of appetite, violent yawning, severe sneezing, tearing, weakness, depression, nausea, vomiting, intestinal spasms, and diarrhea.

Heart rate and blood pressure become elevated. Chills alternate with flushing, excessive sweating, and waves of gooseflesh. The skin resembles that of a plucked turkey, the basis of the expression "cold turkey" to signify abrupt withdrawal without treatment. Abdominal cramps and pains in the bones and muscles of the back and extremities are also characteristic, as are muscle spasms and kicking movements that may be the basis for the expression "kicking the habit."

Other signs of withdrawal include ejaculations in men and orgasms in women. The failure to take foods and fluids, combined with vomiting, sweating, and diarrhea, results in marked weight loss and dehydration. Occasionally there is cardiovascular collapse.

At any point in the course of withdrawal the administration of a suitable opiate will completely and dramatically suppress the symptoms of withdrawal. Without treatment, opiate withdrawal runs its course and most of the severe symptoms disappear in seven to ten days, but it takes six months or more for the body to return to normal.

Long-Term Withdrawal— The Vicious Cycle of Craving and Relapse

Even though a drug has completely left the brain as well as the body, its effects may linger for a very long time. Recognition of this is critical for an understanding of the problem

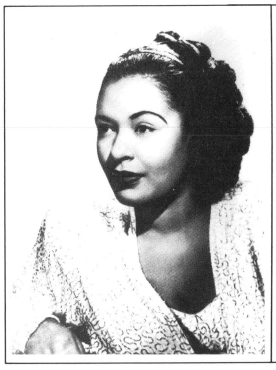

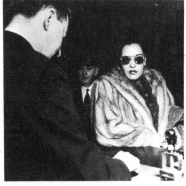

During the 1930s and 1940s jazz and blues singer Billy Holiday (left, and during an arrest, below) was addicted to heroin, and in and out of jail and detox hospitals. On May 25, 1959, she collapsed. At first left unattended in a private facility, she was transferred to a Harlem hospital, where she died.

of opiate addiction. Once the initial phase of withdrawal is complete, and the severe and agonizing period of "cold turkey" has passed, the addict is by no means free of the effects of withdrawal. Instead, there follows a second and prolonged phase of withdrawal whereby the addict is over-whelmed with corrosive feelings of despair and worthlessness, depression, the inability to tolerate stress or pressure, and intense waves of craving for heroin. The craving comes as an overpowering desire for relief from the unbearable psy-chic pain. It is not that one is searching for the "high" but rather he or she is filled with a desperate longing to be restored to normal, to end the unrelenting torment of de-pression and hopelessness. All too often the result is drug-seeking behavior, a relapse to heroin use, re-addiction, and a return to a life of procuring a regular supply of heroin and doing whatever is necessary to support the habit.

Detoxification—Kicking Heroin the Old Way

Until the 1960s the only medically approved technique for treating heroin addicts was a medical treatment called detoxification. Addicts were admitted to a special federal or state hospital where over a period of several weeks their daily dose of opiates was gradually lowered until they were

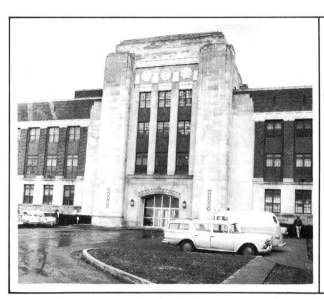

Initially, the "cure" for heroin addicts consisted of a gradual weaning from all drugs, during which the users were often switched to other drugs, such as methadone. Generally it included a stay at a hospital such as this federal detox facility in Kentucky. Unfortunately, upon leaving most returned to a life of drugs.

completely drug-free, or detoxified. Typically they were switched from morphine or heroin to methadone and then detoxified from methadone. This was done because, though withdrawal from methadone lasted somewhat longer, it appeared to be less painful than from heroin or morphine. When detoxification was complete, patients were discharged and sent home.

Unfortunately, detoxification was a miserable failure— after leaving the hospital more than 90% of the patients relapsed to opiate use. Those who did not die on the streets remained trapped within the cycle of addiction-detoxification-relapse. Without a doubt, opiate addiction was a chronic disease. No matter how many times an addict was detoxified, the cycle continued unbroken.

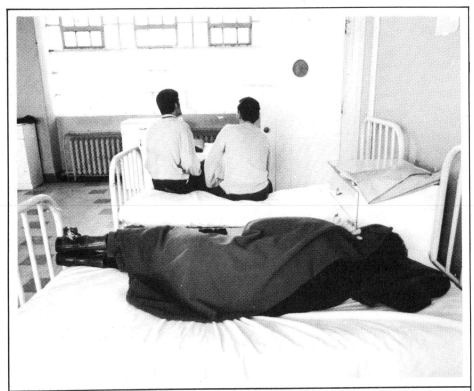

Three new patients at a neuro-psychiatric institute in New York relax in the detoxification section before starting on the methadone maintenance program. With the introduction of methadone, the addict was given the hope that one day he or she could live a normal life.

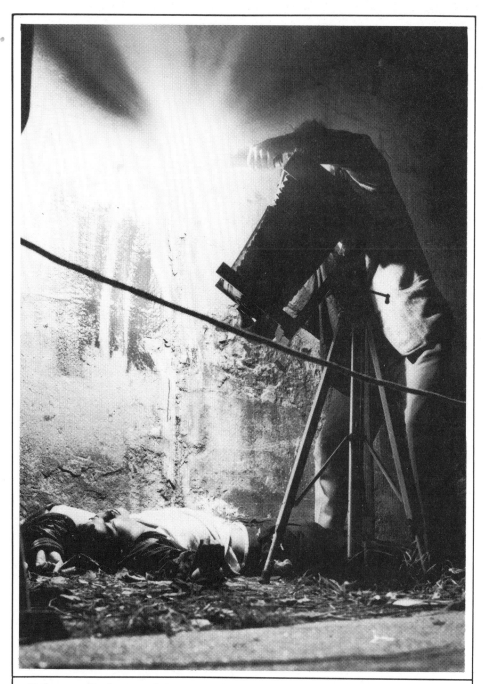

Before methadone maintenance programs, most addicts were trapped within the cycle of addiction-detoxification-relapse. Photographs such as this were used to dramatize the fate of the addict, but they had little effect. Addiction was too complex for such a simple approach.

CHAPTER 3

METHADONE: A NEW CHOICE, A NEW HOPE

*T*he term narcotic has traditionally been used to refer to a particular group of drugs that produced effects similar to morphine—sleep or a state of stupor. Popular usage, especially in the media and when used in reference to drug legislation and law enforcement, has weakened the term. Now, regardless of its relationship to opiates, any substance that either sedates, has a depressive effect, or causes dependence is often referred to as a narcotic. At one time, even cocaine, a stimulant, was mislabeled a narcotic in federal legislation. Because it has become so imprecise and ambiguous in scientific circles, the term narcotic has generally become obsolete and has been substituted with the term opiate.

Methadone and Other Opiate Drugs

The opiates represent a class of drugs of which morphine, heroin, and methadone are members because of their common origin, chemistry, and effects. Crude opium is obtained from the milky juice contained in the unripe seed capsule of the poppy plant. The juice is dried to a brownish gummy mass, and then is made into a powder which contains a number of alkaloids, a specific class of organic chemicals. Chief among these alkaloids are morphine and codeine.

Morphine is the standard against which all other drugs that have morphine-like effects, whether derived from crude opium or synthesized from chemicals, are compared. These drugs are referred to as the opiate analgesics. (The term analgesic or analgesia refers to the reduction or elimination of pain.) However, in addition to their analgesic properties, they produce other strong effects which imbue them with a high potential for abuse, or what is referred to as abuse liability.

Codeine is commonly used as a cough suppressant in cough medicines, or combined with aspirin for relief of minor pain. Compared with morphine it is much less potent, and thus is not the preferred drug of addicts.

Heroin, first introduced in 1898, is derived from morphine and produces virtually identical effects. Possibly because it enters the brain more readily than morphine, and thereby produces more potent effects, it is the major drug of choice among opiate addicts. It has been tested as a

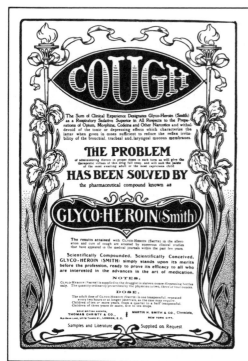

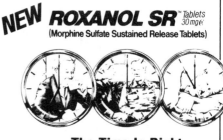

The Time Is Right

Soon after its discovery in 1898 heroin was included in medications such as this cough suppressant, and its abuse potential was largely ignored. Today drugs that contain morphine, such as Roxanol SR, used to combat the severe pain associated with cancer, are highly controlled.

treatment for severe and intractable pain, particularly among terminally ill cancer patients, and is still widely used in Great Britain for this purpose. However, it has no general use in medical practice in the United States.

Meperidine was first synthesized in 1939, and is derived not from crude opium powder but from laboratory chemicals. With effects very similar to morphine's, it has wide medical use for the treatment of relatively severe pain. Because it is so commonly used to ease pain in post-surgical patients, it has become well known, but by its trade name, *Demerol.* Though it is difficult to obtain meperidine through illicit channels, it has a very high abuse liability.

Methadone, a completely synthetic opiate, was first synthesized by German chemists during World War II and used as an analgesic. Chemically it is quite different from morphine, but it produces effects that are nearly identical. Though it was introduced as a maintenance treatment in 1945, the value of methadone in the detoxification of heroin addicts was first recognized in the 1950s, following the study of its pharmacology in the United States. While it is being used more frequently in the treatment of pain associated with terminal cancer, over the past two decades its major use has

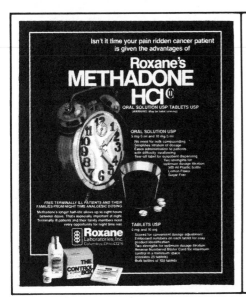

Because methadone's pain-killing effects are long-lasting, it has proven to be beneficial as an analgesic for terminally ill cancer patients, providing continuous relief. Methadone use does lead to addiction, but in some cases this is preferable to unceasing, excruciating pain.

been for the treatment of heroin addicts. Though available on the street as a relatively cheap alternative to heroin, it tends to be used only if heroin is unavailable.

Discovering the Benefits of Methadone

In 1964 Drs. Vincent Dole and Marie Nyswander began a study at Rockefeller University which evolved, quite unexpectedly, into a totally new approach to the treatment of the opiate addict. Over a period of a year they studied six heroin addicts who had volunteered to live in a research ward at a New York City hospital. The study was designed to measure, over a long-term period, their metabolic, physiological, and biochemical characteristics as they lived in the well-controlled research environment. It was previously determined that the subjects were in good health, and during the experiment they were given a well-regulated diet. Known amounts of morphine were dispensed regularly and thus the addicts did not have to steal or evade the police to acquire the drug. In addition, they had no access to alcohol or other illicit drugs. Dole and Nyswander hoped to determine whether there might be some physiological characteristics of addicts which would explain their addiction and high rate of relapse. They thought that addicts might have some sort of metabolic disease whereby to function normally their body "needs" opiates, the same way a diabetic needs insulin.

It was found that while the patients were receiving their eight daily doses of morphine and undergoing regular testing, they rapidly escalated in tolerance, were agitated, and demanded progressive increases in dosage. The researchers' inability to hold the patients in even a minimal state of contentment within the ideal and nonpunitive conditions showed the failure of the heroin maintenance scheme. It became obvious that a drug with a longer period of action was needed.

The researchers planned to collect sufficient scientific data while the subjects were receiving injections of morphine, then substitute oral doses of methadone and study the subjects for a similar period of time. Finally the subjects would be detoxified prior to being discharged from the study. However, during the second, methadone, phase of the study, Dole and Nyswander observed something totally unexpected. Rather than languishing passively on the ward, as the subjects had done while receiving morphine injections, when switched to oral methadone they became normal, well-adjusted, effectively functioning human beings. In addition, it appeared that they had lost their craving for heroin.

For example, one of the patients in the study was a 21-year-old man of Irish background who had been addicted to heroin since the age of 14. He had dropped out of school at 15 and subsequently served two prison terms for narcotics violations. While being maintained on methadone, he earned a high-school equivalency diploma. He went on to earn a full college scholarship, graduate with a degree in aeronautical engineering, and after six years on methadone began work on a master's degree.

While other success stories were nowhere near as dramatic (though since 1965 thousands of patients have had comparable rehabilitations), they did create hope for what

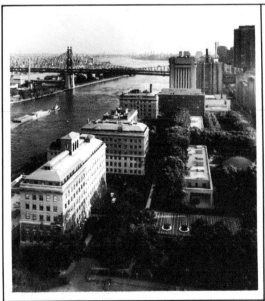
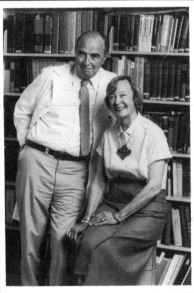

A view of Rockefeller University where Drs. Marie Nyswander and Vincent Dole conducted a study of heroin addicts which unexpectedly led to the development of the methadone maintenance program.

had been a totally hopeless problem. The outlook seemed promising indeed. For the first time in years, former addicts got off the detox-relapse merry-go-round and began leading relatively normal and productive lives free of crime and illicit drug use.

In 1965, in the *Journal of the American Medical Association,* Dole and Nyswander published preliminary findings on their first 22 patients. All were male, aged 19 to 37, and with a history of several years of heroin addiction with relapse after detoxification. Upon entering the study they were immediately stabilized on oral methadone while they lived in an unlocked hospital ward. The exact procedure for weaning patients from street heroin onto methadone was to evolve during the course of this and subsequent studies. The results were described by Dr. Dole and his co-workers in a 1968 issue of the *Journal of the American Medical Association:*

> *The new patient should be given methadone in relatively small divided doses, for example, 10 mg (milligrams) twice daily, and brought to maintenance level (80 mg to 120 mg per day) gradually, over a period of four to six weeks. Some experience in the regulation of dose is necessary: if the medication is increased too rapidly, the patient will become over-sedated during the first few weeks, and may experience urinary retention and constipation; whereas if the dose is inadequate, a patient who has been using a large amount of heroin will have unnecessary withdrawal symptoms.*
>
> *As the dose is gradually increased over a period of four to six weeks, the medication makes the patient refractory [unresponsive] to narcotic drugs and eliminates (or greatly reduces) any narcotic drug hunger, presumably by maintaining a blockade of the sites of narcotic drug action. There should be no euphoria or other undesirable side effects (except mild constipation) if the medication is given in proper dosage. If the patient appears to be sedated during this induction phase the dose of methadone should be held constant or reduced until further tolerance is developed.*

During methadone treatment the patients were given a complete and thorough medical and psychiatric evaluation, and their family, housing, and employment statuses were reviewed. After the first week and for the following six weeks, if accompanied by a staff member, they could leave the ward to attend school, shop, or go to a movie. During this hospitalization phase the staff emphasized the reduction of the generally high anxiety level of the patients and provided each with individualized attention. (In subsequent years of the study this hospitalization phase would be eliminated, and the entire treatment, including initial stabilization on methadone, would be done on an outpatient basis.)

"Narcotic Hunger" Disappears

During the next phase of the study, the patients left the hospital and returned home, continuing the study as outpatients. Upon their daily return to the hospital they were required to drink their medication in the presence of a

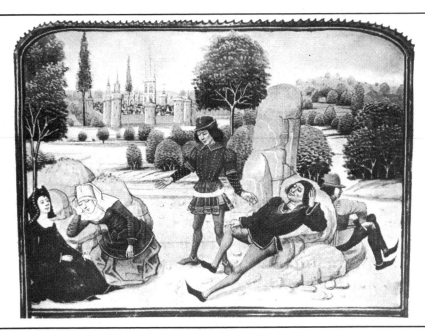

Morpheus distributing sleep and dreams in a 15th-century miniature painting used to illustrate a book by Christiane de Pisan (1363-1432), reputed to be the first professional female writer.

clinic nurse (methadone was typically mixed in the fruit-drink Tang) and to provide a urine sample. It was necessary for the nurse to ensure that patients actually took their methadone, rather than diverting it to the street for illicit sale. The urine samples were analyzed for the illicit use of heroin.

The final phase of treatment marked the major goal of the project—the complete social rehabilitation of the addict whereby he or she would become socially normalized and self-supporting. The most dramatic effect of treatment, Dole and Nyswander reported, was the disappearance of "narcotic hunger." They pointed out that prior to the methadone program all of the patients had previously attempted to remain drug-free after they had gone through standard de-toxification treatment. But after discharge their craving for heroin had always returned, especially overpowering under conditions of stress. On methadone maintenance, however, opiate craving never occurred. The patients claimed that they could be with heroin addicts—even watch them inject

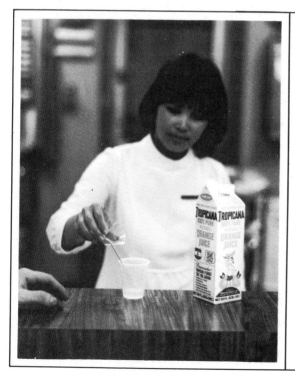

Because methadone is generally dispensed only at clinics and in liquid form, authorities thought that its use could be controlled and that thus it would be difficult for an addict to divert the drug into the black market. However, some patients were clever. They would leave the clinics with the liquid still in their mouths and outside spit it into sponges or containers.

heroin—and could now tolerate frustrating situations, which in the past would have led to heroin use. Results of the urine analyses verified that heroin use was rare and sporadic.

Another important finding described by Dole and Nyswander was that patients on methadone maintenance were unable to get high on injected heroin, either when administered as part of the hospital study or when acquired on the street. Four of the 22 patients admitted to "shooting" heroin with friends. Much to these patients' surprise, not only did they fail to experience euphoria or the usual "rush," but they had no reaction whatsoever. Thus, methadone appeared to act as a block against the heroin high, and as a result discouraged illicit use.

The only medical complication repeatedly observed was constipation—a problem easily remedied with a laxative or an occasional enema. No other medical problems appeared. It was reported that mental and neuromuscular functions were normal—the patients exhibited no deficiencies on a standard motor coordination test. Patients performed well in school and on the job. All in all, Dole and Nyswander were unable to find any medical or pyschological test that could distinguish the methadone subjects from normal control subjects.

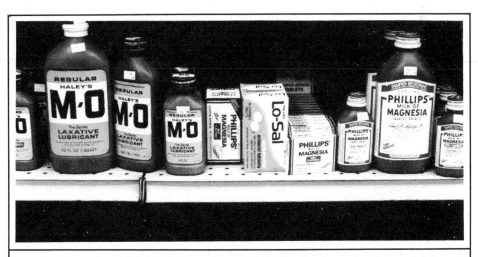

Initially methadone's side effects seemed limited to constipation, which can be easily alleviated by laxatives. However, other reactions such as cardiac arrest, insomnia, and skin rashes have been observed.

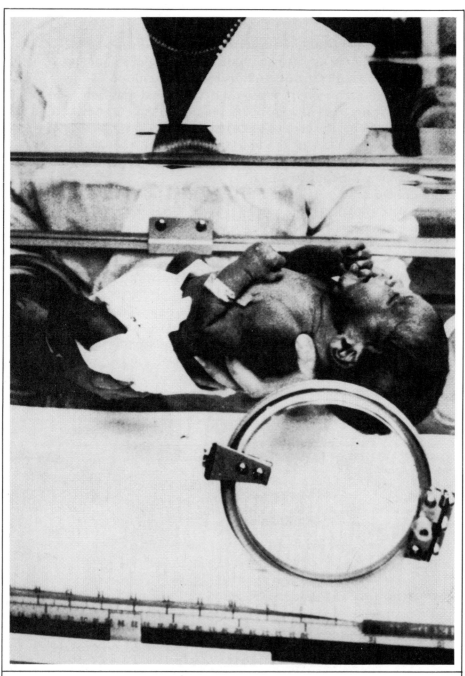

Both heroin and methadone readily pass from a pregnant woman to the fetus. Thus, when an expectant mother abuses either of these drugs she is creating an addiction for two persons. Here, a two-day-old infant, born to an opiate addict, suffers from withdrawal symptoms.

CHAPTER 4

THE EFFECT OF HEROIN AND METHADONE ON PREGNANCY

*A*pproximately one-half of the women addicted to heroin report reduced sex drive and sexual activity, as well as abnormal or complete cessation of menstrual function. Once on methadone maintenance, most women regain normal menstruation, sex drive, and sexual activity. Of the heroin users who remain fertile, and of the majority of women who enter methadone programs, many become pregnant and have children.

Dangers to the Infant

There are two things which can be asserted with relative certainty about the use of either heroin or methadone during pregnancy. Firstly, when used during pregnancy none of the opiate drugs, including heroin and methadone, have been shown to produce birth defects in babies. Birth defects refer to such abnormalities as cleft lip, cleft palate, missing or extra fingers, or deformities of the arms and legs. But secondly, when these same drugs are taken during pregnancy, the baby becomes just as addicted, or, more precisely, as physically dependent, as the mother. Therefore, when the infant is born and thus removed from its supply of opiates which it received from the mother, soon after birth it will go through opiate withdrawal. The symptoms include jerky movements, nearly continuous, high-pitched crying, irritability, and disturbed eating and sleeping patterns. If the symptoms are very severe or persist over several days or weeks, in many cases the baby will need to be medicated with a tranquilizer or other suitable drug. Although the withdrawal symptoms slowly subside over several weeks, some infants remain restless and hyperactive, and for as long as four to six months continue to have difficulty sleeping. Some children exposed to opiates during pregnancy exhibit what is called "short attention span," a syndrome which may persist at least until the time of entering school. However, it is not known whether or not there are long-term behavioral or psychological effects that persist beyond childhood.

The pregnant addict presents an especially difficult treatment problem. Ideally, the unborn child should not be exposed to *any* drugs during pregnancy, but even non-addicted pregnant women frequently have some sort of medical problem—for example, infection, high blood pressure, or morning sickness—which requires treatment with a prescription drug. The opiate addict who becomes pregnant while in methadone treatment is already taking a powerful medication. If her pregnancy is detected within the first two months, she might have the option of detoxifying from methadone, with the understanding that if methadone withdrawal is too severe, she can immediately go back on methadone. If she is beyond the third month, detoxification is *not*

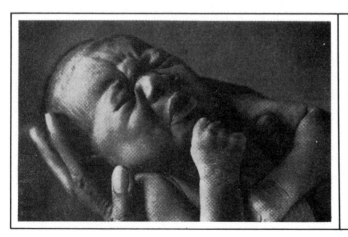

Withdrawal symptoms in the four-day-old addict may include hyperactivity, screaming, and irritability. Sadly, as children these "ex-addicts" may suffer from a short attention span.

recommended because both the fetus and the mother are likely to undergo withdrawal, which is very dangerous, greatly increasing the possibility that the baby will die in the womb and creating a health risk to the mother.

If the mother decides to remain on methadone—and most do—another difficult problem arises. Should she remain on a high dose of 60 mg–80 mg, or should her daily maintenance dose be reduced to 10 mg–30 mg? The high dose would probably produce more severe withdrawal in the infant after birth, while a lower dose might reduce the likelihood of severe symptoms and ultimately be better for the health of the baby.

As will be discussed later, with a low maintenance dose there is the increased probability that the patient, because the dose fails to "hold" her, will either leave the program and go back out on the street or remain in the program, supplementing her methadone with illicit heroin.

This presents a terrible dilemma for the clinic staff members who are attempting to provide the best treatment for *two* patients—the mother and her unborn baby. If the mother is kept on a high dose, her baby will be forced to risk the most severe symptoms; but if the dose is lowered, the mother often resorts to using illicit heroin which, in turn, puts her baby at risk.

Treating the Mother

Nearly all clinics have opted for a low maintenance dose, and the available data has borne out the fear that many of these patients do, in fact, increase their use of street drugs. More distressing is one doctor's observation that when a group of pregnant addicts supplemented their low maintenance dose with drugs they acquired on the street, they had a higher total drug intake than heroin addicts who were *not* in a methadone program.

There is no simple and direct approach to the treatment of the pregnant addict. One can only hope for the development of improved techniques that provide optimum treatment for the mother with a minimum risk to her baby. But unfortunately there is presently no indication that such a solution is forthcoming. Because of this, each year thousands of infants will be born who, without choice, have been needlessly exposed to dangerous drugs.

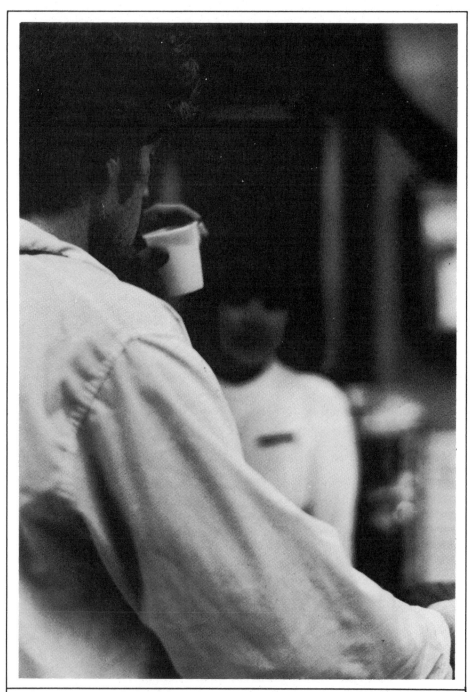

As the number of methadone clinics increased so did criticism of the whole maintenance program. One question was frequently asked: Was addiction to one drug better than addiction to another?

CHAPTER 5

A CLOSER LOOK AT METHADONE MAINTENANCE

*G*iven the dismal history of failure of previous attempts to treat opiate addicts, why did methadone produce results which appeared nothing short of miraculous? If opiate addiction were a simple problem, a simple solution might have been anticipated. But the issue is not whether we should use cold water or put butter on a minor burn, or if it is appropriate to take extra vitamin C to treat a cold. We are trying to find a *safe* and *effective* treatment for a major disease that up until now had no cure. In this instance safe means assurance that both short- and long-term use of methadone does not produce any serious medical risk. And effective means that treatment does indeed rehabilitate the addict so that he or she no longer uses illicit opiates and can lead a reasonably crime-free life.

Because a methadone maintenance program involves the use of public funds—both state and federal—the safety and effectiveness of the treatment had to be proven to convince those entrusted with those funds that the program can be successful. Some critics felt that methadone maintenance was nothing more than giving free dope to dope fiends—like giving free gin to alcoholics—and so it was necessary to demonstrate the effectiveness and benefit of the program to both the addict and the public.

There is no question that the Dole and Nyswander methadone experiment produced positive and encouraging results, but what was not clear was just what aspect of the treatment was responsible for the favorable outcome. Does methadone produce an effect on the brain different from heroin's? And to what extent does all the special attention given the patient by the physicians, nurses, and social workers contribute to positive results? These and other questions must be answered in order to arrive at a better understanding of how methadone maintenance works.

Clearly there must be features of methadone that are important for the treatment's success. Firstly, unlike heroin or morphine, methadone is effective when taken orally, thus obviating the need for trained personnel to make up sterile solutions (as is necessary for all drug injections), to search for usable veins (after repeated injections it becomes difficult to penetrate a vein), or to keep track of the stock of sterile syringes and needles. Secondly, methadone stays in the body much longer and thus is effective for a longer period. A single dose of heroin "holds" an addict for only

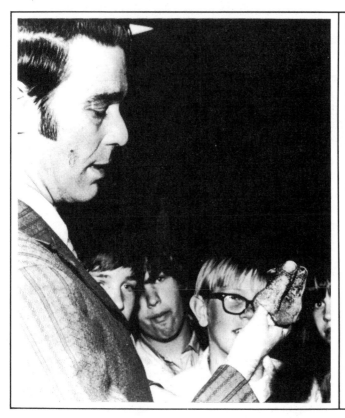

Often ex-addicts become active opponents to drug use. Here a former 15-year heroin addict, at one of his stops during a tour of Oregon, displays the result of repeatedly injecting the drug into his wrist—a mummified hand.

about four hours—six at most—after which he or she begins to experience withdrawal and exhibits drug-searching behavior. By comparison, methadone remains effective for about 24 hours, and so rather than six daily injections of morphine, only one oral dose of methadone is needed. Thus the heroin addict is relieved of the ceaseless euphoria-withdrawal cycle which repeats itself every few hours. And finally, it appeared that the relatively high dose of methadone effectively blocked the opiate high if the addict again injected heroin. However, in order to get more precise and reliable answers, the study needed to be repeated on a much larger scale.

Methadone Is Put to the Test

Dole and Nyswander arranged with the New York City Commissioner of Hospitals to expand the project to include a much larger number of addicts. In addition, an independent evaluation unit headed by Dr. Frances Gearing was established at The Columbia University School of Public Health. By December 1973 the methadone maintenance program, which ten years before had started with six volunteers, now included approximately 40,000 patients. In 1974 Dr. Gearing published a report entitled "Methadone maintenance treatment five years later—Where are they now?" The evaluation included the first 1,230 patients admitted to the methadone program between 1964 and 1968.

All of the patients had been volunteers and had to meet the following criteria to be admitted to the program:

- a resident of metropolitan New York
- at least 20 years of age (later lowered to 18)
- without obvious psychiatric symptoms
- addicted to heroin for at least five years
- a record of arrests/incarceration
- a record of previous treatment failures

The 1,230 patients were characterized as 85% men and 15% women; 40% white, 40% black, and 20% Hispanic; and with an average age of 33.7 years. The average number of years addicted was eight, and all the patients had records of previous criminal activity and were thus characterized as "hard-core" or "criminal" addicts. The program focused on the patients' social rehabilitation, emphasizing eventual employment by enabling them to complete their formal education, to learn a vocational skill, or both.

To provide an objective measure of success in the program, three criteria were used: (1) an increase in social productivity, determined by looking at employment, schooling, or vocational training; (2) a decrease in antisocial behavior, measured by comparing any reports of arrest or time spent in jail with the subject's previous record; and (3) increased self-esteem and the desire to succeed, judged by the subject's recognition of and willingness to accept help for excessive use of alcohol and/or other drugs, and/or psychiatric problems.

Results of the Five-Year Study

In 1973, the end of the five-year study period, among the original 1,230 patients 770 were still under observation. During that period 460 patients (37%) left the program. Of

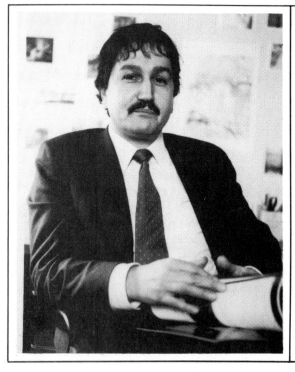

Despite criticism of the methadone maintenance program and the reports of adverse side effects, success stories are not rare. David Patterson (left), who in 1985 had been using methadone for 15 years, is a successful New York lawyer.

the 770 patients remaining in treatment, there was an increase in employment from 36% to 72%. Moreover, of those who became employed the trend was for individuals to become upwardly mobile—advancing from unskilled to semi-skilled, from semi-skilled to skilled, and from sales and clerical to professional and managerial. Dr. Gearing described that in general "the type of job which a man on methadone maintenance is most likely to hold is one involving technical and motor skills—such as motor mechanic, TV or air-conditioning repairman, truck or cab driver, tool and die worker, printer, computer or TV technician. Among the women, the majority are employed as waitresses, beauticians, switchboard operators, IBM operators, typists, or secretaries, with a few practical nurses, technicians, models, and dancers."

In the 770 patients who continued in treatment, criminal activity decreased substantially. Since starting the program 654 (85%) had no record of arrests, whereas 116 persons were arrested, some more than once. However, comparison with the patients' previous arrest record for the

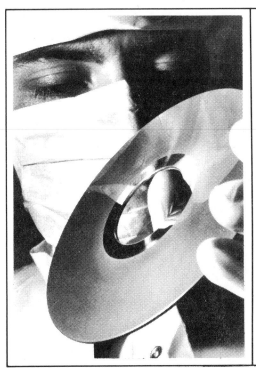

Dole and Nyswander's five-year study of addicts in a methadone maintenance program concluded that, for the 63% who remained under observation, employment increased from 36% to 72%. Some were able to hold down jobs as computer technicians, such as this person inspecting a computer data storage disk.

three years prior to the program shows a decrease of from 201 arrests per 100 persons to only 1.24 arrests per 100 persons.

For about 25% of the patients, chronic overuse of alcohol, barbiturates, and amphetamines, alone or in combination with other drugs, a syndrome which existed previous to methadone treatment, continued to be a problem. For a significant number of patients this interfered with their ability to obtain or hold a job. Dr. Gearing reported that "continued problems with drug abuse and alcohol, despite valiant efforts on the part of the treatment teams, have been responsible for the majority of the discharges.... Alcohol and drug abuse have also been involved in a substantial proportion of the deaths, both while in treatment and after leaving the program." However, despite researchers' fear that methadone's effective blocking of the heroin euphoria might *lead* to the abuse of other substances, this occurred only rarely. Clearly the abuse of *all* substances had to be treated.

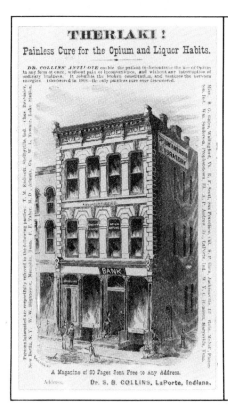

In 1873 Dr. S. B. Collins advertised *Theriaki, his "Painless Cure for the Opium and Liquor Habits," as a panacea for drug problems, but it was unsuccessful. In 1973 a 5-year follow-up study showed that 25% of the methadone-using patients exhibited chronic overuse of alcohol, barbiturates, and amphetamines—a polydrug syndrome that probably existed prior to beginning methadone use.*

Fifty-one patients, less than 7% of the 770, elected to detoxify completely from methadone, and an equal number went to low maintenance doses (30 mg or less per day) with the hope that they could eventually become methadone-free. Of these, 23 (18%) were unable to tolerate being drug-free or continue on a low maintenance dose, and they subsequently returned to high-dose methadone maintenance.

There were 393 patients who left the program and were not in treatment by the end of the study period. Forty-one percent of these had been arrested or imprisoned at least once, 27% had been repeatedly hospitalized for detoxification, 15% were in a drug-free program, 3% were being treated by a private physician, and 6% were known to have died. Of the 393, 11% came in and out of the program and were considered "revolving door" patients.

Although these results did not satisfy the high expectations and optimism of the initial study, they seemed to indicate that methadone maintenance did help rehabilitate a significant number of hard-core heroin addicts, most of whom had previously tried other forms of treatment, yet without success. A high percentage remained in treatment, stopped using illicit drugs, and became productive, law-abiding citizens. But also, as Dole and Nyswander were to caution, methadone maintenance, as part of a supportive program, facilitates social rehabilitation but clearly does not prevent opiate abuse after the addict leaves the program. Nor does social rehabilitation guarantee freedom from relapse. However, there now seemed to be some hope for the hopeless.

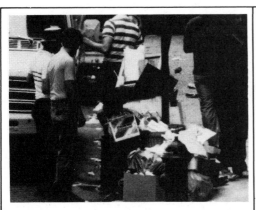

Methadone treatment is not successful for everyone. Some people return to the streets and combine methadone with other drugs, and every year deaths due to toxic combinations are reported. One man, who sold part of his methadone supply to buy wine, barbiturates, and heroin, died from a methadone-heroin combination.

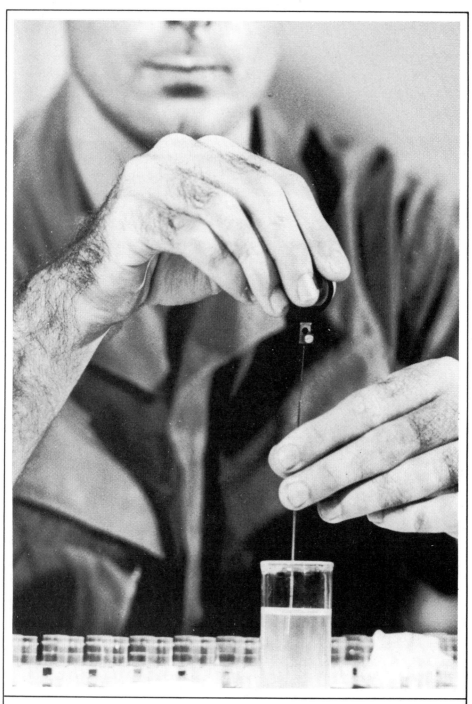

Before leaving Vietnam, soldiers' urine was tested for opiates by lab technicians using a special, sophisticated, $26,000 machine.

CHAPTER 6

THE "NEW SOLUTION" SPREADS

Many questions about the specifics of methadone maintenance remained unanswered. For example: Is it necessary to use such a high dose of methadone (100 mg–120 mg) or would a low maintenance dose of 20 mg–40 mg per day be just as effective? What is the effect of long-term use of methadone on an individual's ability to remain drug-free after detoxification from methadone? Might group psychotherapy serve some useful role as part of the overall treatment to prevent dropping out or illicit drug use? Can we determine why so many fail and use this information to improve their prognosis? Can we identify those individuals who are more likely to benefit from treatment? What was needed was a concerted effort, guided and supported by the National Institute on Drug Abuse, to provide better research data.

While answers to these and other pressing questions were still being sought, methadone maintenance programs spread rapidly across the country. In the late 1960s some 3,000 heroin addicts were receiving methadone in medically supervised programs. In 1971 a program was initiated to maintain some 20,000 addicts in New York State alone, and by 1972 there were 275 licensed methadone programs throughout the United States. By the mid 1970s there were somewhere between 70,000 and 80,000 individuals in methadone programs, a figure that remains relatively unchanged in 1985.

Solution or Illusion?

As methadone maintenance spread, controversy over the program grew, and spirited opposition came from all fronts—the medical professionals, law enforcement officials, politicians, religious and community leaders, journalists, writers, and scientists. Many remained unconvinced of the effectiveness of the program. Some contended that it was perpetuating rather than solving the opiate problem. There were accusations that it amounted to no less than genocide against the poor blacks and Hispanics who made up the vast majority of addicts seeking help. And some complained that energy and resources were being diverted away from drug-free programs run by ex-addicts, programs that, unlike the cold-turkey detoxification hospitals of the 1950s, were claiming success in getting addicts both socially rehabilitated and drug-free.

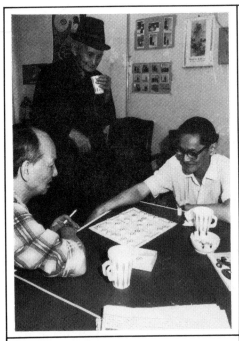 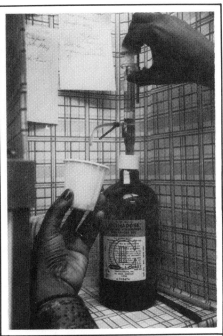

Yee (standing), 86 years old and a drug user since he was 11, is a patient in a methadone maintenance program for Chinese addicts.

The Food and Drug Administration requires that methadone, when used in maintenance therapy, be dispensed by approved programs.

Of those in the medical community who seriously questioned the methadone maintenance program, none were as vehemently opposed and outspoken as Drs. Henry Lennard, Leon Epstein, and Mitchell Rosenthal. In 1972 they co-authored a paper entitled "The Methadone Illusion," which appeared in the highly respected and prestigious journal *Science.* They faulted the basic assumptions proposed by Dole and Nyswander and set off a lively and heated debate.

For example, as to the "blockade" effect of methadone, they suggested that:

> ... this phenomenon is produced by administering high daily doses of the drug. ... With this high dosage, the body is probably not affected by smaller, additional amounts of heroin. A sufficiently massive dose of heroin, however, will still override this "blockade" and produce experiential effects. It should also be added that methadone does not establish cross-tolerance with the nonopiate drugs, such as stimulants, barbiturates, and alcohol; it has been noted that these drugs seem to be used by a sizable number of methadone maintenance patients to gain the euphoria otherwise denied them. In a recent study of 40 methadone maintenance patients, ... it was found that 82% of the patients had used at least one detectable drug ...; 77% of the total group had used heroin concurrently with methadone; 30% used barbiturates; and 25% used amphetamines.

As to the claim that there are virtually no side effects from methadone, the authors asserted that when comparing

> ... the performance and everyday behavior of methadone maintenance patients with that of non-drugged individuals or with "drug-free" ex-addicts, many observers report that addicts who are maintained on methadone are somewhat somnolent (i.e. sleepy) tire more easily, and require more sleep than do nondrugged individuals. Their reflex actions are somewhat abnormal. They frequently perspire more profusely and are often constipated. Sexual impotence also occurs, especially in older men.

They further felt that the proponents of methadone maintenance revealed

> ... *a lack of appreciation of those very factors that initially propelled an individual into taking drugs. Such a comparison between reliance on drugs and reliance on persons overlooks the obvious fact that few, if any, persons are ever "on their own," that we are all dependent on people, that we are sustained and shaped through the support of our family, friends, and co-workers, and, indeed, through the social networks and associations in which we are located. In the case of the addict, such social arrangements have often been deficient and incomplete. He has, in the past, been unable to be dependent upon other human beings.*

Among their strongest statements was the following assertion:

> *Methadone appears, for several reasons, to offer a medical and scientific solution that makes it respectable. It appears to give important results at low cost in the great public concern about addiction-related crime (results in the form of reduced crime and arrest rates for addicts participating in the program). However, the methadone approach does not touch the roots of the drug problem, which are inextricably bound up with current social arrangements and inequities; with the glorification of technology, and especially of drugs. Methadone permits the illusion of a solution.*

These were strong accusations, indeed, and they would not go unnoticed or unchallenged. In a 1973 issue of *Science*, several letters expressing strong disagreement were published. For example, one doctor could not understand how the authors seemed to treat as insignificant the finding "that methadone treatment has enabled thousands of heroin addicts to move out of lives of degradation, crime, and risk of serious illness and death," and he added that the symptoms of sweating, sleep problems, impotence, and the like may occur early in treatment but do not persist in the long run. Moreover, he pointed out that the authors had ignored published scientific data from their own laboratory which showed that reaction time, motor coordination, alertness, and intellectual functioning were "in the normal range in patients stabilized on methadone." Finally, he made the point that methadone was a treatment specifically for heroin addiction and would not be expected to have any effect on nonopiate drug use.

Dr. Robert Marcus of New York City noted that even though one of the authors of the article was the director of the drug-free program Phoenix House, there was no description of what success that program had had in rehabilitating heroin addicts. He went on to say that the authors

> ... *seem determined that the addict must be helped in the special way that is of particular interest and importance to them. The religious fervor of their article makes it clear that no report of favorable results with methadone would alter their antidrug dogma. This dogma appears to be more important to the authors than either the well-being of the community or of the addict.*

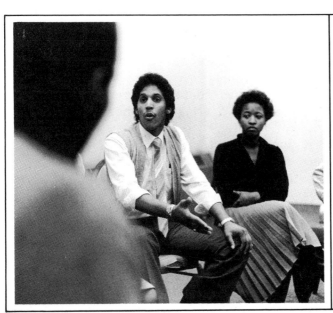

In 1967 five ex-addicts banded together to help each other stay free from drugs. As more people joined, the group eventually formed Phoenix House, a drug-free rehabilitation center. Their self-help encounter sessions have aided thousands of people.

The addiction problem is going to be with us
for a long time and we cannot wait for a panacea
that will be the perfect answer. Not all addicts have
the same needs or similar motivation. There is plenty
of room in the drug treatment field for a broad
spectrum of treatment programs. Scientific study of
these possible programs can only be hampered by
moralistic arguments and an antidrug crusade.

The "Methadone Mills"

In the early 1970s heroin addiction was viewed as a
major domestic menace, and there was pressure directly from
the White House to declare an all-out war on the problem.
Understandably, attention was focused on quickly developing an effective treatment program and providing needed
services to as many heroin addicts as possible throughout
the United States. In the rush to establish methadone programs, a number of changes occurred in the programs which
would only intensify the growing storm of protest over
methadone.

The majority of methadone programs in the large metropolitan areas were privately operated and had little supervision and management by public health officials. Often they
flagrantly disregarded federal and state regulations. Too many
of the directors of these new methadone centers were far
more interested in tapping public funds than in treating
heroin addicts. Gone was the philosophy of Dole and
Nyswander that placed great importance on social rehabilitation as an integral part of methadone maintenance. Many
of the private programs lacked a caring staff concerned with
getting clients back into the mainstream of society where
they could lead productive lives—finish high school, gain
vocational training, and acquire new skills. And the staffs
failed to screen out hard-core criminals, psychopaths, con
artists, and hustlers—many of whom had no intention of
becoming drug-free, but instead were looking for a free
supply of opiates, a fast fix, or a place to hang out and "do
business."

At public hearings these "methadone mills," as the clinics were known, were decried by patients as well as by
residents of the neighborhoods in which the clinics were
located. Residents complained bitterly that some of the pa-

tients loitered noisily on the streets, harassed passersby and deliverymen, and urinated and defecated in public. Mere mention of opening a new methadone clinic now brought a firestorm of protest. Patients complained that the clinics were nothing more than methadone dispensaries that did nothing to help addicts rehabilitate their lives, and that the urinalyses performed to determine illicit drug use were frequently inaccurate. Because of this, some clients not using illicit drugs would be wrongly accused of having "dirty" urine. Mutual contempt and mistrust prevailed, and feelings of discouragement and futility grew among both patients and staff.

The Solution Becomes the Problem

The rapid proliferation of methadone clinics also created a situation in which the use and distribution of methadone were not adequately controlled in many treatment programs. As a result, significant quantities of methadone found their way into the illicit drug market, an occurrence which had a number of serious consequences. For the first time methadone abuse and death due to its overdose began to

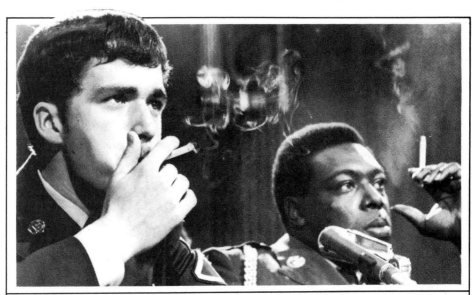

In 1970 two Vietnam veterans, graduates of a military drug treatment facility, told about using marijuana during combat and heroin at home.

emerge as a problem. A number of individuals had been identified with primary methadone addiction, that is, they had become addicted to illicit methadone prior to addiction to heroin or other opiates. (Despite the critics' search for a large population of primary methadone addicts, very few individuals have been discovered.) In addition, there was an increase in deaths due to methadone overdose, as well as accidental poisoning of children. And it had become evident that the clients in the methadone programs were the primary source of methadone diverted to and sold on the street.

In a 1975 issue of *Psychiatry*, Drs. Agar and Stephans, in their article "The Methadone Street Scene: The Addict's View," claimed that methadone diversion typically occurred in two ways. Methadone could be obtained at the time of administration in the clinic by the patient holding the methadone-juice mixture in the mouth until leaving the clinic, and then outside spitting it into a cup, bottle, or sponge. As sickening as it seems, methadone diverted in this manner was actually sold on the street. The more frequent method of diversion, however, was the sale of take-home doses. A convenience to the patients, and a dramatic change from the earlier days of maintenance programs, patients who were considered reliable were given take-home sup-

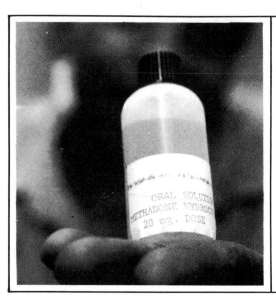

In 1971 this 20-mg dose of methadone was used in the Veterans Administration Hospital drug program. Since then, studies have shown that when doses less than about 50 mg are used patients are more likely either to drop out of the maintenance program or supplement their doses with illicit street heroin.

plies of the liquid methadone for weekends or days when it was inconvenient to visit the clinic. These doses were commonly in the range of 100 mg to 160 mg per day. Many patients were indeed reliable and were grateful not to have to travel a great distance by public transportation seven days a week. Some, however, did sell as much as half or more of their prescribed dose. But how could a patient sell half of his or her dose without experiencing withdrawal? There were three answers:

Firstly, some patients who had take-home doses put themselves on their own self-maintenance programs. They reduced the amount of methadone they ingested and sold the remainder. Sometimes their lowered methadone doses were supplemented with other drugs purchased on the streets, though other times no special technique of coping with withdrawal was necessary because withdrawal did not occur or occurred only minimally. The addicts interviewed said that methadone was potent enough so that the proportion of the dose retained by the patient was usually sufficient to "hold" him for a day or two. Thus the addict could sell part of the maintenance dose with little fear that he or she would become sick.

In short, some patients were obtaining doses that were too high, which allowed them to divert a significant amount for street sale. Once identified, the diversion problem was to have a direct impact on methadone programs, not only with respect to security measures at the clinics, but also with respect to the consideration of the daily dose. Doses

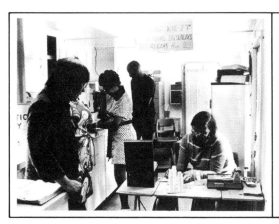

In an attempt to reach as many drug addicts as possible, methadone-dispensing clinics were made more accessible. Here a treatment facility, housed in a trailer, is parked within the community it serves.

were lowered to a maximum of 60 mg–80 mg per day, and take-home privileges were made much more stringent, so that methadone could not leave the clinic in the hands of unstable or untrustworthy patients. In addition, many of the "methadone mills" were shut down. The overall result was a significant drop in both the amount of illicit methadone reaching the street and the occurrence of methadone overdose.

There was, however, one positive result which followed the appearance of street methadone. A considerable number of heroin addicts used the illicit drug to limit their heroin habit or even to establish their own maintenance programs. Considering the fact that in 1985 there is no room for additional patients in methadone clinics, and that applicants are being sent back to the streets to wait for openings, illicit methadone use may not be a bad option for the desperate addict.

A Ten-Year Perspective

In 1976, some 10 years after they had reported on the successful use of methadone to treat a small group of heroin addicts, Dole and Nyswander wrote an appraisal of methadone maintenance, published in the *Journal of the American Medical Association*. In it they reviewed a host of problems that, in their opinion, had seriously hampered the methadone maintenance approach to heroin addiction.

Dole and Nyswander felt that, despite the early success of the program, they had been overly optimistic as to what could actually be accomplished. They were surprised by the fierce and widespread opposition to the notion of treating drug addicts by substituting another drug. And they sadly pointed out that the vast majority of heroin addicts remained on the streets, in part because the methadone programs had lost their ability to attract them into treatment. Dole and Nyswander explained that distributing methadone to a relatively small population, as they had done in their initial study, was quite workable and easy to supervise. However, distribution on a large-scale basis to hundreds of patients proved to be unmanageable because the necessary vigilance and individual attention diminished significantly as the clinic population increased.

Their major complaint was about how highly politicized the field of addiction had become, claiming that now the programs had to adapt to rigid controls established by federal and state agencies. While this did result in closing badly managed programs, it also created a situation in which teams of inspectors were repeatedly combing records in search of technical violations. This policing of the maintenance centers often left the physician and staff defensive and demoralized. Dole and Nyswander concluded with an unhappy view of the future:

> *Methadone and other medication can be produced in large quantity, but the compassion and skillful counseling needed for rehabilitation of addicts are not replicated in the climate of bureaucracy. As in other areas of medical practice, the question is not how many "treatment slots" are available (to use the federal terminology), but what quality of treatment the patients receive. Bureaucratic control of methadone programs has given us "slots," a rule book, and an army of inspectors, but relatively little rehabilitation.*

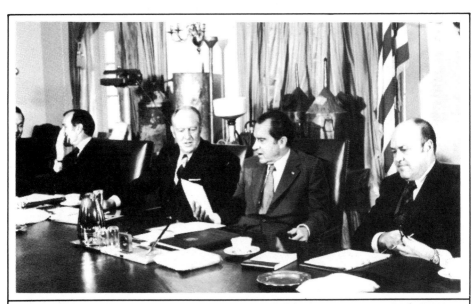

President Nixon in 1972 holding a package of heroin valued at $160,000. Behind him is a still found in Laos, where it was used to refine the drug.

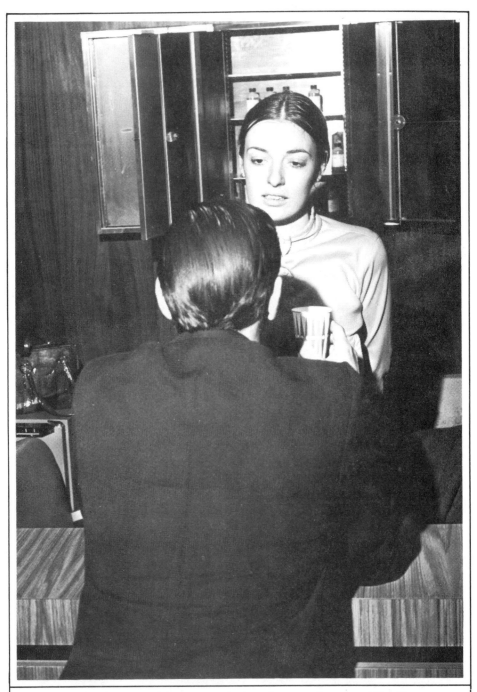

When methadone-dispensing restrictions became lax, complications occurred. In one case a 5-year-old boy mistakenly drank a glass of orange juice that contained methadone and died after going into a coma.

CHAPTER 7

LEARNING FROM THE PAST

By the mid 1980s literally thousands of heroin addicts have been treated in a large number of research programs attempting to answer the many questions about methadone. Since the first studies of Dole and Nyswander, over 275 scientific papers have been published and a great deal of new knowledge has accumulated. However, many critical questions remain unanswered and considerable controversy and disagreement still prevail. Even for the most basic issues there is often no consensus, and for virtually every point of view or opinion there is another that is in disagreement.

The major issues in methadone maintenance include dosage, side effects, treatment duration, client characteristics, and program procedures. And from these issues and the desire to provide the most effective treatment, the following questions arise: Should the dose of methadone be high or low? Are there side effects? How long should a patient remain in a methadone program? Is a certain type of client more likely to benefit from treatment? And, are there certain characteristics of treatment programs that are important for rehabilitation?

Low Dose, High Dose—Is There a Difference?

Of all the methadone maintenance issues, the problem of dosage, especially in methadone clinics with a low-dose philosophy and a focus on detoxification, is among the most

Table 1

Federal Drug Law Enforcement—Summary of Expenditures (Millions of Dollars)					
AGENCY	1981	1982	1983	1984	1985
Dept. of Justice	340.5	377.4	513.8	582.9	600.8
Treasury Dept.	176.7	238.0	293.8	339.0	315.4
Dept. of State	28.4	42.5	47.2	50.2	67.0
Dept. of Transportation	159.1	194.2	218.2	134.8	245.2
Dept. of Agriculture (Research)	1.4	1.4	1.4	1.4	1.4
Forest Service	0.0	0.0	1.0	1.3	1.2
Food and Drug Adm.	1.4	0.8	0.7	0.7	0.7
TOTAL	707.6	854.3	1076.1	1210.3	1221.7

SOURCE: Adapted from the 1984 National Strategy for prevention of Drug Abuse and Drug Trafficking; published by Drug Abuse Policy Office

critical and controversial. For nearly all medication there is a low-to-high dose range that has been determined to be both safe and effective. A dose that is too low fails to produce the desired effects, and a dose that is too high may produce unwanted or toxic side effects. For example, for the relief of minor pain it is recommended that adults take two aspirin tablets. If only a quarter or a half tablet were taken, the dose would likely be too low and little if any pain relief would result. If an amount significantly above the recommended dose were taken, adverse side effects such as headache, dizziness, ringing in the ears, and even death might result.

But in the case of methadone, the dosage problem is complicated by its characteristic opiate tolerance. With repeated administration of methadone, individuals develop tolerance so that increasingly larger doses are required to produce the desired effect. In the initial Dole and Nyswander studies patients were stabilized on 80 mg–120 mg of methadone per day. What occurred, however, was that after patients were stabilized at the maintenance dose, they would begin to feel that they were developing tolerance and prevail upon the clinic staff to raise their dose. Invariably, a power struggle ensued between patients and staff, whereby the patients would claim that the methadone was not "holding" them—that they were beginning to experience with-

Table 2

Federal Drug Abuse Prevention and Treatment Programs—Summary of Expenditures (Millions of Dollars)					
AGENCY	1981	1982	1983	1984	1985
Dept. of Health and Human Services	289.4	178.1	69.7	63.6	78.2
Dept. of Defense	33.6	57.6	69.7	78.8	82.8
Dept. of Justice	4.7	4.4	5.8	9.7	6.8
Dept. of Education	14.0	12.7	2.1	3.0	2.9
Dept. of Agriculture	0.3	0.3	0.3	0.2	0.2
Dept. of Transportation	1.2	1.5	2.5	7.1	5.0
Employment and Training Adm., Dept. of Labor	3.4	1.2	0.4	0.8	0.3
ACTION	2.5	6.8	6.9	6.8	6.9
Veterans Adm.	55.2	55.8	65.1	67.7	69.7
Office of Policy Development, Drug Abuse Policy Office	0.2	0.2	0.2	0.2	0.2
TOTAL	404.4	318.5	222.6	229.5	252.9

SOURCE: Adapted from the 1984 National Strategy for prevention of Drug Abuse and Drug Trafficking; published by Drug Abuse Policy Office

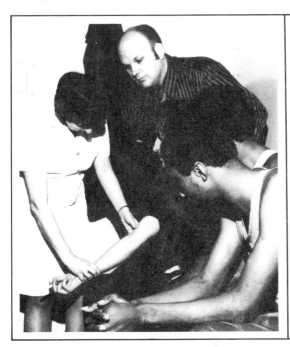

As a nurse examines a prisoner's arm for needle marks, John Goode (standing), chief jail warden at a Jacksonville, Florida, prison, enlists ex-addicts to help new prisoners withdraw from drugs. In addition, at clubs and at shopping-center booths the ex-addicts relate the dangers of substance abuse to the public.

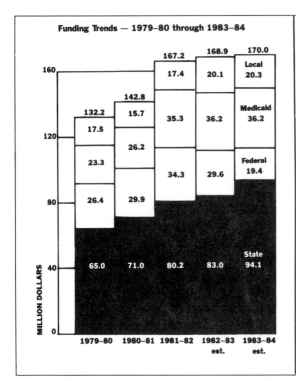

Funding Trends — 1979–80 through 1983–84

	1979–80	1980–81	1981–82	1982–83 est.	1983–84 est.
Total	132.2	142.8	167.2	168.9	170.0
Local	17.5	15.7	17.4	20.1	20.3
Medicaid	23.3	26.2	35.3	36.2	36.2
Federal	26.4	29.9	34.3	29.6	19.4
State	65.0	71.0	80.2	83.0	94.1

MILLION DOLLARS

Figure 2. *Trends in local, state, federal, and Medicaid funding to the New York State Division of Substance Abuse. Although drug use has risen dramatically since 1978, especially among high school students, in recent years the federal government has substantially reduced its support of a variety of drug programs.*

SOURCE: NY State Divisional Substance Abuse *Five Year Plan*, published 1983.

drawal. The threat, explicit or implicit, was that if they continued to feel sick and became abstinent, and the staff refused to increase their dose, they would have no choice but to go out on the street and shoot heroin. If the staff gave in, the scenario would only be repeated again some days or weeks later. The result was that there was virtually no upper limit to the dose that the patients *thought* they needed in order to avoid withdrawal symptoms.

Two factors complicated the issue The patients knew exactly what dose they were receiving. And whether they were actually feeling sick or not was a matter of their word against the staff's. It was possible that patients thought they *ought* to be sick because they had already made up their minds that the dose was too small. Therefore, they did in fact feel sick—a self-fulfilling prophecy.

The problem was finally solved as a result of several clinical studies in which various doses of methadone, ranging from low to high, were given to heroin addicts. In order to eliminate patient bias as to what they thought was an adequate dose, they were not told what dose they were actually receiving. These studies clearly showed that doses around 80 mg were adequate to "hold" most patients, and that generally patients were unable to tell the difference between 80 mg and doses that were as high as 180 mg.

The results of the studies made it possible to develop a policy which set an upper limit to the dose administered in the maintenance programs. In addition, the studies also determined that the actual lower limit, below which the patients did, in fact, begin to get sick, was around 30 mg–40 mg. However, patients on a dose of less than 50 mg were more likely to either drop out of the program or to supplement their methadone dose with illicit heroin. The current policy on methadone dosage, held by a majority of clinicians in the field, is that a dosage of about 80 mg, with a lower limit of 50 mg and an upper limit of 100 mg, is suitable for most patients.

New Studies, New Side Effects

Although the early studies failed to reveal any long-term side effects more serious than sweating and constipation, more thorough research has found methadone to be not quite as problem-free as was originally thought.

One study, which followed several patients maintained on 100 mg of methadone, found a persistent decrease in both pulse and respiratory rate and an increase in rectal temperature. The patients showed increased social withdrawal and lethargy, decreased motivation, reduced efficiency, and a diminished sense of well-being. And they also complained of illness that could not be medically verified. Sexual activity also decreased, and while some improvement occurred over time, the patients constantly complained about problems with sexual potency and delayed ejaculation.

One doctor reported a depression in levels of the male sex hormone testosterone, especially among patients at maintenance doses of 60 mg or higher. In another study there was an observed reduction in the amount of ejaculate, in testosterone levels, and in sperm motility, symptoms often associated with impaired fertility. This occurred at all the maintenance doses studied, though function does appear to return to normal once the individual detoxifies from methadone or other opiates.

However, other studies of patients stabilized on constant daily doses for at least six months discovered no decrease in pulse, respiratory rate, or testosterone levels. Clearly, further objective research is required to more accurately determine methadone's side effects.

Is Treatment Forever?

Dr. Avram Goldstein, one of the leading experts in the field of addiction and methadone maintenance, has pointed out that it has been very difficult to carry out an adequate study of treatment duration. Guided by extensive clinical and research experience, he has suggested that the principal goals in the use of methadone should be to help opiate addicts (a) give up their addiction to illicit opiates; (b) become rehabilitated in society; and (c) eventually give up their dependence on methadone. Furthermore, he assumes that it is better to be maintained on methadone than to be addicted to heroin. Considering this, Dr. Goldstein concludes:

> *1. Patients should be encouraged to detoxify from methadone maintenance and to try abstinence when, in their own opinion, and with the agreement of the clinic staff, they have made sufficient progress in their rehabilitation;*
>
> *2. Patients should be assisted in detoxifying from methadone if they insist, even against staff advice, and whether or not the staff thinks they will be successful;*
>
> *3. Patients should never be compelled to detoxify from methadone against their own wishes, except for disciplinary reasons when the program will be jeopardized by retaining them in the program;*
>
> *4. Former patients who relapse to heroin use after a drug-free period should be able to return, on demand, without delay, and without impediments being placed in their way, for further methadone treatment.*

Who Does Better, Who Does Worse?

Studies of patient characteristics have attempted to go beyond the general observation that a significant number of opiate-dependent patients show significant improvement during methadone treatment. Instead they ask if there are certain types of clients that respond more favorably to treatment than others. After reviewing over 100 studies that examined this problem, the following conclusions can be made:

The factors of age, marital status, and race appear to have some relationship to both whether or not patients remained in treatment and how well they performed. There seemed to be a greater degree of success with those older than 25, nonwhite, and either married or in a stable relationship. Sex and educational background were of little significance. In addition, those who entered the program with a good work history, and who were either skilled or semi-skilled, were more likely to remain in treatment.

Two factors that tended to be associated with patients who had difficulty staying in treatment were criminal history and mental illness. With respect to the latter, those individuals who had a combination of symptoms such as anxiety, depression, and thought disorder were more likely

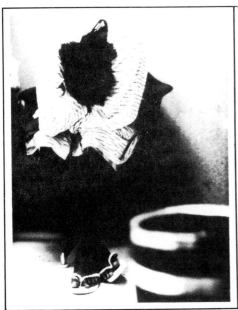

The rate of success of the methadone maintenance program is frequently measured by how long a patient remains in treatment. In addition, patients with certain characteristics are more apt to persist or give up. For example, an individual exhibiting a psychological illness, such as this woman, is more susceptible to failure.

to drop out of treatment sooner. In other words, the more severe the patient's psychological problem, the less likely he or she would remain in treatment.

It must be emphasized that one should not give too much weight to these generalizations. They reflect only trends which *suggest* the sorts of individuals who are more or less likely to benefit from treatment. They should not be taken as hard and fast rules.

Methadone and Job Performance

Data collected over a period of many years strongly indicate that individuals stabilized on methadone maintenance can function on the job as well as normal employees. Although it is difficult to collect hard scientific data, vocational services that have had a long-term experience with maintenance clients report that these persons can hold down an amazing variety of highly skilled and demanding jobs in the workplace. In many instances the employers neither knew nor suspected that the individuals were taking methadone. However, one must keep in mind that the majority of clients who enter methadone programs have never acquired high-level vocational skills, and thus these observations are based on a relatively small number of individuals.

One study showed that of methadone clients who had been hired as cab drivers there was no higher incidence of absenteeism, turnover, or poor productivity than among drivers not involved with drugs.

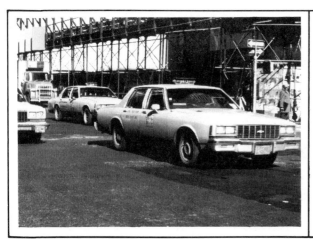

Studies that have measured the ability of an ex-addict to function normally in a drug-free environment have produced many encouraging results. One such study of cab drivers in treatment showed that job performance was not at all affected by the continued use of methadone.

Are Some Treatment Programs Better than Others?

Other studies have dealt with the services related to rehabilitation, including counseling, psychotherapy, family therapy, and social work. These studies are especially important for determining if there are specific characteristics of various treatment approaches that are directly associated with positive results.

It is important to understand that though heroin addicts share the common trait of repetitive, compulsive drug use, they are an extremely diverse group of individuals with regard to their psychological makeup, background, and personal circumstance. For example, in one study of 750 addicts, 85% had been diagnosed as having some degree of psychiatric illness. The most common disorders were depression, antisocial personality, and alcoholism. However, in other ways they were quite diverse: some were single and some were married, some had children, some were employed and some were unemployed, some were about to go to jail while others had just gotten out. Clearly a variety of approaches is required in order to meet the needs of the diverse group of addicts. However, very little good data are available that bear on the issue.

In most programs a major portion of the treatment is carried out by drug counselors, and one would assume that they play an absolutely essential role in the rehabilitation process. Among their numerous responsibilities, they must be aware of the methadone dose, write letters to court, intervene in any personal crises that may arise, explain the rules and routine of the clinic, evaluate patient requests for take-home medication, and refer patients to physicians for evaluation of medical or psychiatric problems. In addition, they must monitor urine test results and psychological growth and adjustment, as well as the patient's legal and employment status. And to further complicate the situation, the counselors' backgrounds are as varied as their duties—some are ex-addicts without a high school diploma, whereas others are college graduates.

While it is difficult to imagine how the programs could successfully operate without these essential services, one such program devoid of all counseling exists in Hong Kong. By simply dispensing adequate doses of methadone to former heroin addicts they have been able to reduce illicit drug traffic and crime and facilitate employment. (Detoxification is not a part of this program.) Some researchers have seriously questioned the effectiveness of counseling, the most pessimistic view being that there are no data proving that it adds anything to treatment. However, a more balanced interpretation would be that the services which the counselor provides have not yet been sufficiently defined to allow a meaningful evaluation. And therefore it is premature and unwarranted to conclude that the counselor is unimportant or without effect. In addressing the human element of the treatment program—what is referred to in mental health jargon as the "interpersonal" ingredient—Dr. Avram Goldstein puts it this way:

> *Large differences may be observed between programs employing identical dosage schedules, and it is apparent that for most addicts much more than methadone alone is required to achieve a change of life style, abstinence from illicit drugs, and social rehabilitation. Even on large doses of methadone, patients do not necessarily give up heroin use. The common complaints that "methadone is not holding me" and that "I need more methadone" evidently are not to be taken at face value but require skillful translation. When the*

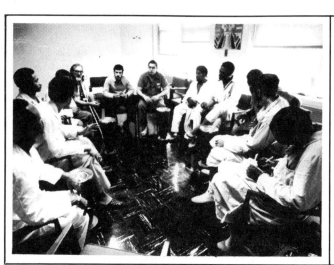

Patients in a Veterans Administration maintenance program discuss what methadone will and will not do for them. Some critics claim that the V.A. does not provide adequate therapy to help patients remain drug-free.

staffs of methadone programs finally accept the fact that such complaints cannot be dealt with succesfully by manipulating the methadone dose, effort can be directed undistractedly toward the interpersonal transactions that are central to the task of rehabilitation.

Whereas counseling focuses on the more specific and practical needs of the patient, psychotherapy attempts to treat the patient's psychological problems. The problem of the effectiveness of psychotherapy is as complex an issue as counseling, and to date the findings are only suggestive and far from conclusive. It can only be said that patients who receive psychotherapy, either as an individual or as part of a family, appear to do better than those who only receive counseling.

In examining all of the research related to various aspects of treatment, including different types of psychotherapy, such as family therapy and relaxation therapy, vocational rehabilitation, and staff training, one can only conclude that there are no clear answers regarding their effectiveness. However, the safest recommendation is for the provision of a variety of services in the clinic, even if only because they are wanted by the clients. The available scientific data, though not conclusive, does suggest that this will provide favorable results.

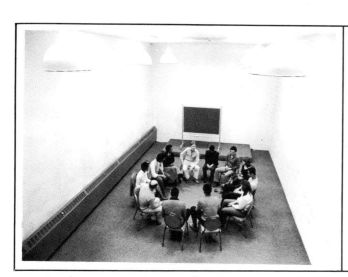

Phoenix House, a strong advocate of drug-free treatment, claims that its residential centers, which use encounter sessions (left) and provide role models to create a supportive environment, help more than 75% of graduates become productive members of society.

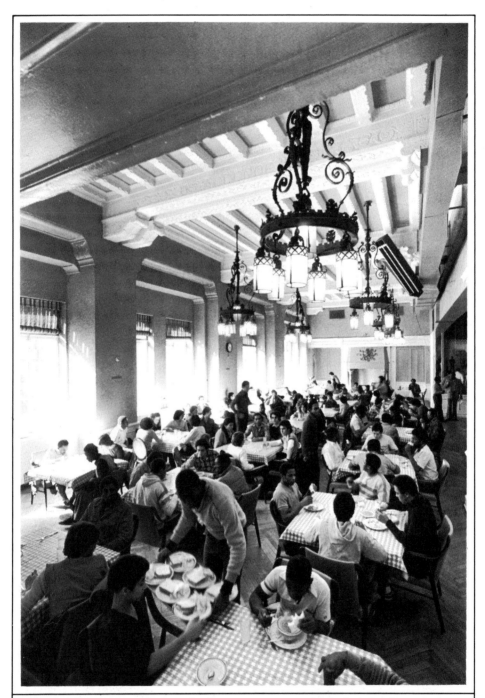

Some critics argue that methadone treatment, which does prolong an addiction and is most frequently administered to blacks, constitutes an insidious form of racial genocide.

CHAPTER 8

ALTERNATIVES TO METHADONE MAINTENANCE

*I*n the past several years there have been some new drugs used in the treatment of heroin addiction. They include the drug *clonidine*, used to relieve the symptoms of withdrawal, *naltrexone*, a type of drug called an opiate antagonist, and *methadyl acetate*, known as LAAM, a long-acting opiate.

The drug clonidine has been used since 1974 for the treatment of high blood pressure, or what is medically called hypertension. In 1978 one doctor reported that clonidine eased the withdrawal symptoms that occur during detoxification from methadone. He studied 11 hospitalized addicts who, after having been on low-dose methadone maintenance, were abruptly taken off their daily dose. When the patients began to show the expected signs of opiate withdrawal, they were administered clonidine. The drug appeared to produce a rapid and dramatic decrease in withdrawal symptoms and psychological distress. This initial report, and several others which followed, raised hopes that a new drug treatment was available that would help those addicts who were attempting to detoxify, and also get them through that critical period of withdrawal when it is so difficult *not* to return to the use of street heroin.

But like other "cures" for opiate addiction, later studies revealed that while the use of clonidine was of some limited usefulness, its safety and effectiveness had yet to be adequately demonstrated. Clonidine can produce dangerous side effects, including severe psychotic and psychiatric symptoms, sedation, sleep disorder, and dangerously low blood pressure.

Initial enthusiasm was based on research which followed too few patients and was carried out under circumstances that posed even more questions. Only further research can determine whether or not clonidine will be of some use in the treatment of withdrawal. But obviously when dealing with the problem of drug addiction one must be suspicious of easy answers.

Naltrexone is considered an *opiate antagonist* because when it is administered it prevents an opiate that is taken soon after from having any effect. It accomplishes this by blocking areas in the brain, called receptor sites, that react to opiates. Moreover, naltrexone produces no effects of which the individual is aware—there are no observable changes in mood or physiological function. This drug has been used to help detoxified opiate addicts from becoming readdicted, even if they return to a life-style or neighborhood where opiates are readily available. The temptation to use any illicit opiate is removed by the action of the antagonist, and thus the addict is entirely opiate-free.

However, naltrexone cannot be used by persons with liver disease, and it is estimated that 60% of all heroin addicts have this disease, often brought on by hepatitis. And because the addict must be highly motivated to insure complete rehabilitation, it is estimated that for only 10%–15% of heroin addicts will naltrexone prove entirely successful. Therefore, like methadone maintenance, some do well with naltrexone treatment while others do not. Although, like clonidine, it has been used in clinics since 1974, it is still an experimental drug and until 1984 had not been available for general clinical use.

LAAM is an experimental drug that is a methadone substitute. It is called a long-acting opiate because it produces opiate-like effects, but compared with heroin, which is broken down in the body very rapidly, or methadone, which "holds" a patient for 24 hours, LAAM remains active for about 48 hours. Thus it can be taken either every other day or on a Monday, Wednesday, Friday schedule. LAAM has been tried with patients who either find it difficult to get to the clinic every day or are susceptible to diversion of take-home methadone. In one study of 74 patients on LAAM treatment, it was found that, after an 11-month period, 72% of the patients were still in treatment. The few patients

90

dissatisfied with LAAM complained about the 72-hour weekend period following the Friday dose. In order to hold them
over the weekend, this dose was somewhat higher than the
Monday or Wednesday dose, and they felt over-medicated
on Friday and under-medicated by Sunday. Aside from these
few patients, however, LAAM appeared to offer a safe and
effective alternative to methadone, especially where methadone diversion is a hazard to public health.

A Drug-Free Home-away-from-Home

There have been a large number of drug-free, therapeutic
rehabilitation programs, but the Phoenix House Foundation
operates one of the largest in the United States. These programs are generally opposed to the use of any drug treatment, such as methadone, to treat a drug problem. They
maintain that drug abuse has its roots in a personality disorder that requires residential therapeutic treatment. Individuals may stay in residence for 14 months or longer before
beginning to reenter life in their own community. The em-
phasis is on group therapy, which makes use of confronta-
tional encounter sessions that are brutally frank and severely
critical in characterizing an individual's attitudes and personality. As in other treatment approaches, however, the
dropout rate has been reported to be as high as 75% during
the first year and 90% before completion of the program.

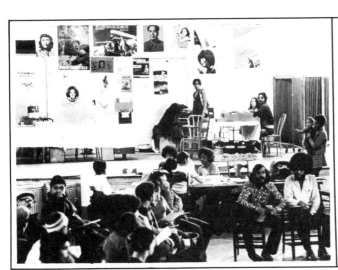

In 1973 at a drug detoxification center at Lincoln Hospital in New York, patients participating in "The People's Program" were offered social action as an alternative to addiction.

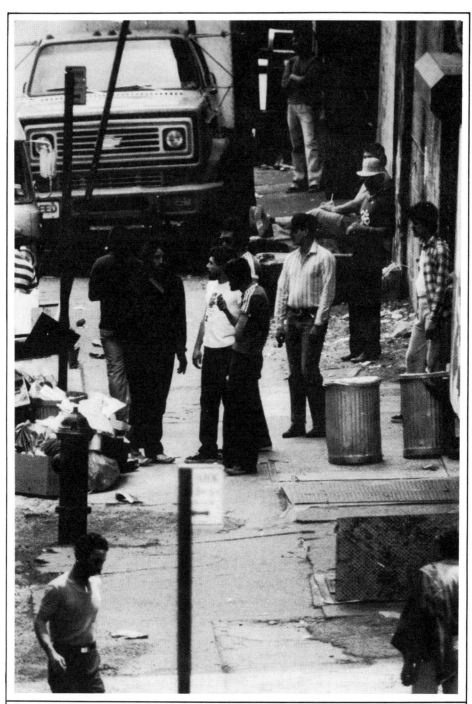

Drug users—even suburban teenagers—travel to New York City's Lower East Side to buy and sell supposedly the best pills, cocaine, and heroin.

CHAPTER 9

THE DILEMMA OF POLYDRUG ABUSE

*I*n the field of addiction research there are two things never in short supply—addicts and theories about how addicts become addicts. Social theories stress the turmoil of adolescence, that tumultuous period between childhood and adulthood when a person seeks a unique identity by being different, yet is terrified of being too different—always fearful of peer disapproval. "Devil-Heroin, be my friend—you tempt me, you dare me but you'll never conquer me—I am Superman, I am Wonderwoman!"

Others stress the degradation of poverty—living with rats, hunger, unemployment, welfare, food stamps, and dehumanization. "Oh God-Heroin, I pray you, set me free!" Or the social theories focus on the unrelenting tension and fierce competition of life in the "fast lane"—the entertainment business, high finance, or moving with the "beautiful people." "Heroin, my Guardian Angel, watch over me, make me cool and lovable, help me win friends and influence people."

Psychological theories talk of the "addictive personality," of the person who seeks immediate and instantaneous gratification. "Sweet-candy-sex-heroin, make it ALL happen NOW!" Psychiatric theories suggest that chronically depressed or anxious individuals seek relief from their mental anguish through opiates. "Tranquilizer-Heroin, please make me stop feeling so bad, so crazy!"

Individual theories that attempt to explain *all* drug addiction will ultimately fail; yet those that focus on smaller, subgroups of individuals are more often accurate, at least superficially. But it remains certain that drug addiction in general, and opiate addiction in particular, is an enormously complex disorder, or more likely, a multitude of disorders with multiple causes—such as social, psychological, and medical. For effective treatment one must locate the root of the causes, and this treatment must also include promoting the education of both teenagers and adults about the hazards of opiate use, alleviating social injustices, and supporting the accurate diagnosis and treatment of mental illness.

However, just as some progress is being made and there seems to be some hope for the opiate addict, a new dilemma surfaces: the opiate addict, the person who once abused only one kind of drug, for which methadone might have been useful, has begun to abuse many different drugs at the same time.

Up through the 1970s, among the major drugs of abuse heroin was abused most often, and the majority of addicts were poor—the lower class, the left-out, the left-behind,

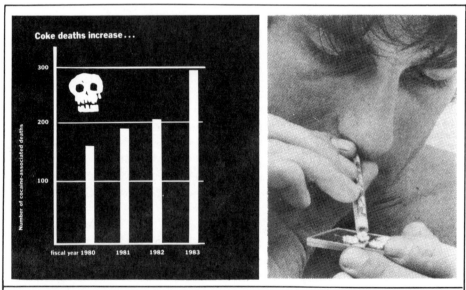

As cocaine use rises—reflected by a threefold increase in use by high-school seniors between 1975 and 1982—so does the number of related deaths.

those who supported their habit with shoplifting, mugging, armed robbery, car theft, prostitution, and drug peddling. Now in the 1980s social class boundaries among drug abusers have all but disappeared, and the original addicts have been joined by a new breed of wealthy, educated, white-collar professionals. Many were raised in the affluent suburbs, attended private schools and Ivy League universities, and are upwardly mobile—moving easily into high-paying jobs in law, finance, high technology, entertainment, or the fashion industry. But heroin now shares its popularity with cocaine, and both are abused not only by the poor, but also by middle-class entrepreneurs and the privileged upper class. And these new addicts may be addicted primarily to either heroin or cocaine, or may use both simultaneously in some endlessly alternating upper-downer, soaring-crashing cycle.

In a series published in *The New York Times*, one expert stated that:

> *What we have is the baby boom generation of post World War II that has shifted from marijuana to cocaine. Many of them get so comfortable with the idea of so-called recreational drugs in the 1960s and 1970s and they are smack dab in the middle of life, dealing with problems they never thought they would have to deal with.*

An example of such an individual is a 29-year-old investment banker who graduated from an Ivy League college and moved to New York City in 1978. After he entered a private rehabilitation program he told the following story:

"Like most people of my generation, I started with pot in high school. I experimented with cocaine in college, but it was too expensive then. When I got to the city, a lot of people in my social and business lives were doing it. It was part of being accepted, like drinking. It was there and I did it along with everyone else. It was a form of release at the end of the day. It didn't trouble me because it was illegal. As long as I wasn't selling it, I didn't feel I was committing a crime.

"The first couple of years, I was snorting two or three grams a week, costing me $200 to $300, but I could afford it. I was making $50,000 in my job and I have a considerable outside income, another $50,000. The people I know are deep into six and seven figure incomes. When you make half a million a year, you can afford a cocaine life-style. After a deal you say, 'Let's celebrate, get a couple of suites in a hotel, girls from an escort service, a couple of limos, a case of Dom Perignon and an ounce of cocaine.' It's just part of that good life.

"In 1982 I had a lot of business pressures. I wanted to leave the company I was with and start my own investment-consulting company. I was unhappy at work and at the time I became friendly with a group of people in the commodities exchange who do it [use drugs] in massive quantities. I stopped buying a gram or two from friends and started to meet with real hard-core dealers. I needed larger and larger quantities—$2,000 a week. I could afford it but it was

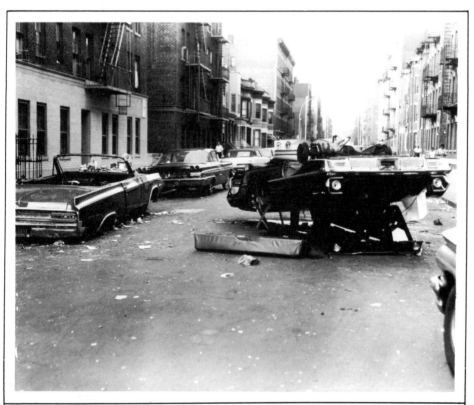

Until the 1980s drug abuse was usually associated with the urban poor. However, in the 1980s the wealthy addict appeared.

hitting my savings, not coming out of my paychecks.

"Last year I got married and there was the pressure of work and a fight with my landlord. Coke put me in a different world. I didn't care anymore. I was going downhill at work. All I was looking forward to was the next high. I thought I was concentrating but I wasn't. I'd go to Lutèce for a business luncheon and not eat a thing. There were a couple of deals that I definitely blew.

"Last October I confessed to my wife I was doing it in large quantities. I went to a psychiatrist and stopped for two months. Then it started again, worse than ever. I felt wired but not in a frenzied condition. My hands shake and you're always blowing your nose; it's like having a chronic cold. I was spending money faster than I was making it. In the last year and a half, it cost me more than $100,000. Emotionally

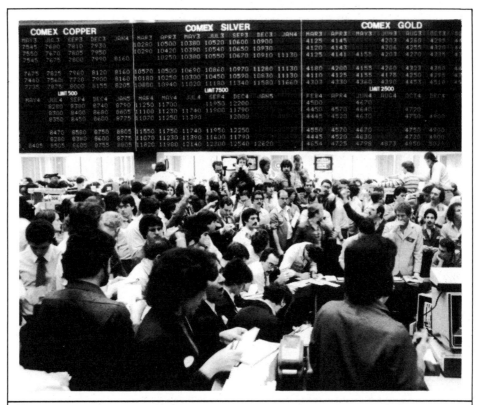

The young executive's acceptance of recreational drug use, the relative affordability of drugs, and corporate pressures have led to polydrug use.

it was tearing me apart. I was losing my temper, losing my shrewdness. I was talking too much when I should have been discreet. I tortured my wife—started fights with her just for the fun of it. Sometimes I was so high I'm lucky I didn't kill myself by stepping in front of a bus."

A New York State study of new heroin users found a large number of people, not unlike this businessman, who said they had turned to heroin in an attempt to relieve the psychological stresses caused by cocaine. The study stated that "they get so wired, so hyperstimulated by chronic cocaine use that they can't sleep or function. They resort to heroin to avoid the depression which normally happens when cocaine is cut off, only to become addicted."

Those who become addicted to drugs are the last to admit that they have a problem. Even when their lives have become totally unmanageable—a total living hell—and they have to face the fact of having lost their job, home, family, and self-respect, they persist in saying "I can stop any time I want." And, indeed, they are right—they stop every day.

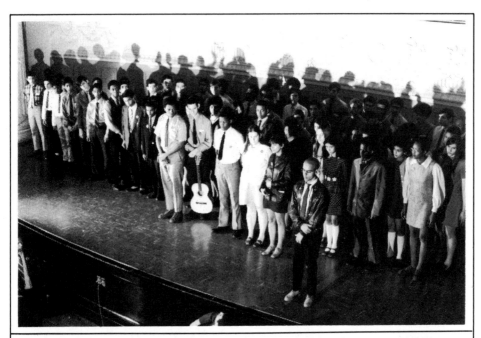

In 1970 these teenagers—all one-time heroin addicts—commemorated New York City youths who had died from drug overdose.

Unfortunately, they also relapse every day. One view of alcoholism, taught by Alcoholics Anonymous but true of all drug addictions, is that addiction is a disease that tells the addict he does not have a disease. So as the world crumbles around him, this fierce denial functions as the major psychological obstacle that keeps the addict on drugs and out of treatment.

Despite the alarming prevalence of this self-denial, it would be a mistake not to acknowledge some advances that have occurred. Among the most important has been the recognition that drug addiction is not simply "the work of the devil," a corruption of morals, or weakness of will, but rather a disease or disorder which can be effectively treated with a variety of medical, psychological, and social interventions. For some, methadone maintenance may be the best long-term choice, whereas for others methadone may be a stepping-stone to detoxification. Many will be helped by drug-free, residential treatment centers, halfway houses, programs such as Narcotics Anonymous, or any combination of these. There is also some comfort in knowing that once addiction and total dependence on a drug is acknowledged, once a person admits that his or her life is out of control and completely unmanageable, there are choices available that can help lead a person back to a drug-free life.

> Look to this day,
> For it is life,
> The very life of life.
> In its brief course lie all
> The realities and verities of existence,
> The bliss of growth, The splendor of
>   action,
> The glory of power—
>
> For yesterday is but a dream,
> And tomorrow is only a vision,
> But today, well lived,
> Makes every yesterday a dream of
>   happiness
> And every tomorrow a vision of hope.
>
> Look well, therefore to this day.

SANSKRIT PROVERB

APPENDIX

STATE AGENCIES
FOR THE PREVENTION AND TREATMENT
OF DRUG ABUSE

ALABAMA
Department of Mental Health
Division of Mental Illness and
  Substance Abuse Community
  Programs
200 Insterstate Park Drive
P.O. Box 3710
Montgomery, AL 36193
(205) 271-9253

ALASKA
Department of Health and Social
  Services
Office of Alcoholism and Drug
  Abuse
Pouch H-05-F
Juneau, AK 99811
(907) 586-6201

ARIZONA
Department of Health Services
Division of Behavioral Health
  Services
Bureau of Community Services
Alcohol Abuse and Alcoholism
  Section
2500 East Van Buren
Phoenix, AZ 85008
(602) 255-1238

Department of Health Services
Division of Behavioral Health
  Services
Bureau of Community Services
Drug Abuse Section
2500 East Van Buren
Phoenix, AZ 85008
(602) 255-1240

ARKANSAS
Department of Human Services
Office on Alcohol and Drug Abuse
  Prevention
1515 West 7th Avenue
Suite 310
Little Rock, AR 72202
(501) 371-2603

CALIFORNIA
Department of Alcohol and Drug
  Abuse
111 Capitol Mall
Sacramento, CA 95814
(916) 445-1940

COLORADO
Department of Health
Alcohol and Drug Abuse Division
4210 East 11th Avenue
Denver, CO 80220
(303) 320-6137

CONNECTICUT
Alcohol and Drug Abuse
  Commission
999 Asylum Avenue
3rd Floor
Hartford, CT 06105
(203) 566-4145

DELAWARE
Division of Mental Health
Bureau of Alcoholism and Drug
  Abuse
1901 North Dupont Highway
Newcastle, DE 19720
(302) 421-6101

DISTRICT OF COLUMBIA
Department of Human Services
Office of Health Planning and
  Development
601 Indiana Avenue, NW
Suite 500
Washington, D.C. 20004
(202) 724-5641

FLORIDA
Department of Health and
  Rehabilitative Services
Alcoholic Rehabilitation Program
1317 Winewood Boulevard
Room 187A
Tallahassee, FL 32301
(904) 488-0396

Department of Health and
  Rehabilitative Services
Drug Abuse Program
1317 Winewood Boulevard
Building 6, Room 155
Tallahassee, FL 32301
(904) 488-0900

GEORGIA
Department of Human Resources
Division of Mental Health and
  Mental Retardation
Alcohol and Drug Section
618 Ponce De Leon Avenue, NE
Atlanta, GA 30365-2101
(404) 894-4785

HAWAII
Department of Health
Mental Health Division
Alcohol and Drug Abuse Branch
1250 Punch Bowl Street
P.O. Box 3378
Honolulu, HI 96801
(808) 548-4280

IDAHO
Department of Health and Welfare
Bureau of Preventive Medicine
Substance Abuse Section
450 West State
Boise, ID 83720
(208) 334-4368

ILLINOIS
Department of Mental Health and
  Developmental Disabilities
Division of Alcoholism
160 North La Salle Street
Room 1500
Chicago, IL 60601
(312) 793-2907

Illinois Dangerous Drugs
  Commission
300 North State Street
Suite 1500
Chicago, IL 60610
(312) 822-9860

INDIANA
Department of Mental Health
Division of Addiction Services
429 North Pennsylvania Street
Indianapolis, IN 46204
(317) 232-7816

IOWA
Department of Substance Abuse
505 5th Avenue
Insurance Exchange Building
Suite 202
Des Moines, IA 50319
(515) 281-3641

KANSAS
Department of Social Rehabilitation
Alcohol and Drug Abuse Services
2700 West 6th Street
Biddle Building
Topeka, KS 66606
(913) 296-3925

KENTUCKY
Cabinet for Human Resources
Department of Health Services
Substance Abuse Branch
275 East Main Street
Frankfort, KY 40601
(502) 564-2880

LOUISIANA
Department of Health and Human
  Resources
Office of Mental Health and
  Substance Abuse
655 North 5th Street
P.O. Box 4049
Baton Rouge, LA 70821
(504) 342-2565

MAINE
Department of Human Services
Office of Alcoholism and Drug
  Abuse Prevention
Bureau of Rehabilitation
32 Winthrop Street
Augusta, ME 04330
(207) 289-2781

MARYLAND
Alcoholism Control Administration
201 West Preston Street
Fourth Floor
Baltimore, MD 21201
(301) 383-2977

State Health Department
Drug Abuse Administration
201 West Preston Street
Baltimore, MD 21201
(301) 383-3312

MASSACHUSETTS
Department of Public Health
Division of Alcoholism
755 Boylston Street
Sixth Floor
Boston, MA 02116
(617) 727-1960

Department of Public Health
Division of Drug Rehabilitation
600 Washington Street
Boston, MA 02114
(617) 727-8617

MICHIGAN
Department of Public Health
Office of Substance Abuse Services
3500 North Logan Street
P.O. Box 30035
Lansing, MI 48909
(517) 373-8603

MINNESOTA
Department of Public Welfare
Chemical Dependency Program
  Division
Centennial Building
658 Cedar Street
4th Floor
Saint Paul, MN 55155
(612) 296-4614

MISSISSIPPI
Department of Mental Health
Division of Alcohol and Drug Abuse
1102 Robert E. Lee Building
Jackson, MS 39201
(601) 359-1297

MISSOURI
Department of Mental Health
Division of Alcoholism and Drug
  Abuse
2002 Missouri Boulevard
P.O. Box 687
Jefferson City, MO 65102
(314) 751-4942

MONTANA
Department of Institutions
Alcohol and Drug Abuse Division
1539 11th Avenue
Helena, MT 59620
(406) 449-2827

NEBRASKA

Department of Public Institutions
Division of Alcoholism and Drug Abuse
801 West Van Dorn Street
P.O. Box 94728
Lincoln, NB 68509
(402) 471-2851, Ext. 415

NEVADA

Department of Human Resources
Bureau of Alcohol and Drug Abuse
505 East King Street
Carson City, NV 89710
(702) 885-4790

NEW HAMPSHIRE

Department of Health and Welfare
Office of Alcohol and Drug Abuse
  Prevention
Hazen Drive
Health and Welfare Building
Concord, NH 03301
(603) 271-4627

NEW JERSEY

Department of Health
Division of Alcoholism
129 East Hanover Street CN 362
Trenton, NJ 08625
(609) 292-8949

Department of Health
Division of Narcotic and Drug Abuse
  Control
129 East Hanover Street CN 362
Trenton, NJ 08625
(609) 292-8949

NEW MEXICO

Health and Environment Department
Behavioral Services Division
Substance Abuse Bureau
725 Saint Michaels Drive
P.O. Box 968
Santa Fe, NM 87503
(505) 984-0020, Ext. 304

NEW YORK

Division of Alcoholism and Alcohol
  Abuse
194 Washington Avenue
Albany, NY 12210
(518) 474-5417

Division of Substance Abuse
  Services
Executive Park South
Box 8200
Albany, NY 12203
(518) 457-7629

NORTH CAROLINA

Department of Human Resources
Division of Mental Health, Mental
  Retardation and Substance Abuse
  Services
Alcohol and Drug Abuse Services
325 North Salisbury Street
Albemarle Building
Raleigh, NC 27611
(919) 733-4670

NORTH DAKOTA

Department of Human Services
Division of Alcoholism and Drug
  Abuse
State Capitol Building
Bismarck, ND 58505
(701) 224-2767

OHIO

Department of Health
Division of Alcoholism
246 North High Street
P.O. Box 118
Columbus, OH 43216
(614) 466-3543

Department of Mental Health
Bureau of Drug Abuse
65 South Front Street
Columbus, OH 43215
(614) 466-9023

OKLAHOMA
Department of Mental Health
Alcohol and Drug Programs
4545 North Lincoln Boulevard
Suite 100 East Terrace
P.O. Box 53277
Oklahoma City, OK 73152
(405) 521-0044

OREGON
Department of Human Resources
Mental Health Division
Office of Programs for Alcohol and
Drug Problems
2575 Bittern Street, NE
Salem, OR 97310
(503) 378-2163

PENNSYLVANIA
Department of Health
Office of Drug and Alcohol
Programs
Commonwealth and Forster Avenues
Health and Welfare Building
P.O. Box 90
Harrisburg, PA 17108
(717) 787-9857

RHODE ISLAND
Department of Mental Health,
Mental Retardation and Hospitals
Division of Substance Abuse
Substance Abuse Administration
Building
Cranston, RI 02920
(401) 464-2091

SOUTH CAROLINA
Commission on Alcohol and Drug
Abuse
3700 Forest Drive
Columbia, SC 29204
(803) 758-2521

SOUTH DAKOTA
Department of Health
Division of Alcohol and Drug Abuse
523 East Capitol, Joe Foss Building
Pierre, SD 57501
(605) 773-4806

TENNESSEE
Department of Mental Health and
Mental Retardation
Alcohol and Drug Abuse Services
505 Deaderick Street
James K. Polk Building, Fourth Floor
Nashville, TN 37219
(615) 741-1921

TEXAS
Commission on Alcoholism
809 Sam Houston State Office Building
Austin, TX 78701
(512) 475-2577

Department of Community Affairs
Drug Abuse Prevention Division
2015 South Interstate Highway 35
P.O. Box 13166
Austin, TX 78711
(512) 443-4100

UTAH
Department of Social Services
Division of Alcoholism and Drugs
150 West North Temple
Suite 350
P.O. Box 2500
Salt Lake City, UT 84110
(801) 533-6532

VERMONT
Agency of Human Services
Department of Social and
Rehabilitation Services
Alcohol and Drug Abuse Division
103 South Main Street
Waterbury, VT 05676
(802) 241-2170

VIRGINIA
Department of Mental Health and
  Mental Retardation
Division of Substance Abuse
109 Governor Street
P.O. Box 1797
Richmond, VA 23214
(804) 786-5313

WASHINGTON
Department of Social and Health
  Service
Bureau of Alcohol and Substance
  Abuse
Office Building—44 W
Olympia, WA 98504
(206) 753-5866

WEST VIRGINIA
Department of Health
Office of Behavioral Health Services
Division on Alcoholism and Drug
  Abuse
1800 Washington Street East
Building 3 Room 451
Charleston, WV 25305
(304) 348-2276

WISCONSIN
Department of Health and Social
  Services
Division of Community Services
Bureau of Community Programs
Alcohol and Other Drug Abuse
  Program Office
1 West Wilson Street
P.O. Box 7851
Madison, WI 53707
(608) 266-2717

WYOMING
Alcohol and Drug Abuse Programs
Hathaway Building
Cheyenne, WY 82002
(307) 777-7115, Ext. 7118

GUAM
Mental Health & Substance Abuse
  Agency
P.O. Box 20999
Guam 96921

PUERTO RICO
Department of Addiction Control
  Services
Alcohol Abuse Programs
P.O. Box B-Y Rio Piedras Station
Rio Piedras, PR 00928
(809) 763-5014

Department of Addiction Control
  Services
Drug Abuse Programs
P.O. Box B-Y Rio Piedras Station
Rio Piedras, PR 00928
(809) 764-8140

VIRGIN ISLANDS
Division of Mental Health,
  Alcoholism & Drug Dependency
  Services
P.O. Box 7329
Saint Thomas, Virgin Islands 00801
(809) 774-7265

AMERICAN SAMOA
LBJ Tropical Medical Center
Department of Mental Health Clinic
Pago Pago, American Samoa 96799

TRUST TERRITORIES
Director of Health Services
Office of the High Commissioner
Saipan, Trust Territories 96950

Further Reading

Brecker, Edward M. and the Editors of Consumer Reports. *Licit & Illicit Drugs.* Boston: Little, Brown and Company, 1972.

Bourne, Peter. *Methadone: Benefits & Shortcomings.* Washington, D.C.: Drug Abuse Council, 1975.

Chambers, Carl D. and Brill, Leon, eds. *Methadone: Experiences & Issues.* New York: Human Sciences Press, 1973.

Danaceau, Paul. *Methadone Maintenance: The Experiences of Four Programs.* Washington, D.C.: Drug Abuse Council, 1973.

Downs, Hunton. *Opium Stratagem.* New York: Bantam, 1973.

Einstein, S. *Methadone Maintenance.* New York: Dekker, Marcel, Inc., 1971.

Hawkins, John A. and Grab, Gerald N., eds. *Opium Addicts & Addiction.* Salem, New York: Ayer Company, 1981.

Glossary

addiction: a condition caused by repeated drug use, including a compulsive urge to continue using the drug, a tendency to increase the dosage, and physiological and/or psychological dependence

alkaloid: any chemical containing nitrogen, carbon, hydrogen, and oxygen, usually occurring in plants

amphetamines: drugs that stimulate the nervous system, generally used as mood elevators, energizers, antidepressants, appetite depressants, and as substances to increase alertness and activity

analgesia: insensitivity to pain without loss of consciousness

analgesic: a drug that produces analgesia

barbiturates: drugs that cause depression of the central nervous system, generally used to reduce anxiety or to induce euphoria

blockade effect: a condition whereby one drug effectively inhibits another drug from producing its usual effects

cardiovascular: of, related to, or involving the heart and blood vessels

clonidine: a drug first used for the treatment of high blood pressure, later found to reduce the withdrawal symptoms associated with methadone detoxification

codeine: a sedative and pain-relieving agent found in opium and related to morphine but less potent

cold turkey: abrupt withdrawal from any drug of addiction without the use of any substance which might ease the withdrawal symptoms

cross-tolerance: a condition of tolerance to one or more drugs caused by the body's tolerance to another drug

detoxification: the process by which an addicted individual is gradually withdrawn from the abused drug, usually under medical supervision and sometimes in conjunction with the administration of other drugs

euphoria: a mental high characterized by a sense of well-being

hepatitis: inflammation of the liver, often associated with the use of contaminated hypodermic needles

heroin: a semisynthetic opiate produced by a chemical modification of morphine

LAAM: methadyl acetate; a long-acting opiate used as a methadone substitute

mainline: to inject a drug intravenously

meperidine: a synthetic drug similar to morphine and used for the treatment of relatively severe pain

metabolize: to convert, by using enzymes, one substance to compounds that can be readily eliminated from the body

methadone: a synthetic opiate producing effects similar to morphine, used to treat pain associated with terminal cancer and in the treatment of heroin addicts

morphine: the principal psychoactive ingredient of opium, producing sleep or a state of stupor, and used as the standard against which all morphine-like drugs are compared

naltrexone: an opiate antagonist, which does not produce dependence or any noticeable effects, though cannot be used by people with liver disease

narcotic: originally, a group of drugs producing effects similar to morphine; often used to refer to any substance that sedates, has a depressive effect, and/or causes dependence

narcotic hunger: a craving for heroin

opiate: a compound from the milky juice of the poppy plant, *Papaver somniferum,* including opium, morphine, codeine, and their derivatives, such as heroin

opiate antagonist: a drug which, when administered, prevents an opiate from having any effect

organic: derived from a living organism and containing carbon and hydrogen

physical dependence: an adaptation of the body to the presence of a drug, such that its absence produces withdrawal symptoms

psychological dependence: a condition in which the drug user craves a drug to maintain a sense of well-being and feels discomfort when deprived of it

refractory: unresponsive; e.g., some claim that methadone makes a patient refractory to heroin and other narcotic drugs *sedative*: a drug that produces calmness, relaxation, and, at high doses, sleep; includes barbiturates

stimulant: any drug that increases brain activity which results in the sensation of greater energy, euphoria, and more alertness

testosterone: a male sex hormone

tolerance: a decrease of susceptibility to the effects of a drug due to its continued administration, resulting in the user's need to increase the drug dosage in order to achieve the effects experienced previously

tranquilizer: a drug that has calming, relaxing effects

withdrawal: the physiological and psychological effects of discontinued usage of a drug

Index